T0249754

Dermatopathology

Guest Editor

STEVEN D. BILLINGS, MD

CLINICS IN LABORATORY MEDICINE

www.labmed.theclinics.com

Consulting Editor
ALAN WELLS, MD, DMSc

June 2011 • Volume 31 • Number 2

SAUNDERS an imprint of ELSEVIER, Inc.

W.B. SAUNDERS COMPANY
A Division of Elsevier Inc.

1600 John F. Kennedy Boulevard • Suite 1800 • Philadelphia, Pennsylvania 19103-2899

http://www.theclinics.com

CLINICS IN LABORATORY MEDICINE Volume 31, Number 2
June 2011 ISSN 0272-2712, ISBN-13: 978-1-4377-2463-9

Editor: Katie Hartner
Developmental Editor: Donald Mumford

Reprints. For copies of 100 or more, of articles in this publication, please contact the Commercial Reprints Department, Elsevier Inc., 360 Park Avenue South, New York, New York 10010-1710. Tel. (212) 633-3813, Fax: (212) 462-1935, E-mail: reprints@elsevier.com.

Clinics in Laboratory Medicine (ISSN 0272-2712) is published quarterly by Elsevier Inc., 360 Park Avenue South, New York, NY 10010-1710. Months of issue are March, June, September, and December. Business and Editorial offices: 1600 John F. Kennedy Blvd., Suite 1800, Philadelphia, PA 19103-2899. Periodicals postage paid at NewYork, NY and additional mailing offices. Subscription prices are $225.00 per year (US individuals), $364.00 per year(US institutions), $120.00(US students), $273.00 per year (Canadian individuals), $460.00 per year (foreign institutions), $165.00 (foreign students). Foreign air speed delivery is included in all Clinics subscription prices. All prices are subject to change without notice. POSTMASTER: Send address changes to *Clinics in Laboratory Medicine*, Elsevier Health Sciences Division, Subscription Customer Service, 3251 Riverport Lane, Maryland Heights, MO 63043. **Customer Service: 1-800-654-2452 (US). From outside of the US and Canada, call 1-314-447-8871. Fax: 1-314-447-8029. E-mail: journalscustomerservice-usa@elsevier.com (for print support) or journalsonlinesupport-usa@elsevier.com (for online support).**

Clinics in Laboratory Medicine is covered in *EMBASE/Exerpta Medica, MEDLINE/PubMed (Index Medicus), Cinahl, Current Contents/Clinical Medicine, BIOSIS and ISI/BIOMED.*

Printed and bound by CPI Group (UK) Ltd, Croydon, CR0 4YY
Transferred to Digital Print 2012

Contributors

CONSULTING EDITOR

ALAN WELLS, MD, DMSc
Department of Pathology, University of Pittsburgh, Pittsburgh, Pennsylvania

GUEST EDITOR

STEVEN D. BILLINGS, MD
Section of Dermatopathology, Anatomic Pathology; Department of Anatomic Pathology, Cleveland Clinic, Cleveland, Ohio

AUTHORS

KLAUS J. BUSAM, MD
Professor of Pathology and Laboratory Medicine, Weill Medical College of Cornell University; Attending Pathologist, Department of Pathology, Memorial Sloan-Kettering Cancer Center, New York

LOREN E. CLARKE, MD
Assistant Professor of Pathology and Dermatology, Departments of Pathology and Dermatology, The Penn State Hershey Medical Center, Hershey, Pennsylvania

PHILIP D. DA FORNO, MBChB, MD, FRCPath
Specialist Registrar, Department of Histopathology, University Hospitals of Leicester NHS Trust, Leicester Royal Infirmary, Leicester, United Kingdom

A. HAFEEZ DIWAN, MD, PhD
Director of Dermatopathology, Departments of Pathology and Dermatology, Baylor College of Medicine; Department of Pathology, University of Texas MD Anderson Cancer Center, Houston, Texas

ANTOINETTE F. HOOD, MD
Professor and Chair, Department of Dermatology, Eastern Virginia Medical School, Norfolk, Virginia

LAINE H. KOCH, MD
Dermatology Resident, Department of Dermatology, Eastern Virginia Medical School, Norfolk, Virginia

ALEXANDER J. LAZAR, MD, PhD
Departments of Pathology and Dermatology; Sarcoma Research Center, The University of Texas MD Anderson Cancer Center, Houston, Texas

ROSSITZA LAZOVA, MD
Associate Professor, Department of Dermatology and Pathology, Yale University School of Medicine, New Haven, Connecticut

ASHLEY R. MASON, MD
Dermatology Resident, Department of Dermatology, Eastern Virginia Medical School, Norfolk, Virginia

TIMOTHY H. MCCALMONT, MD
Professor of Clinical Pathology and Dermatology, Co-Director, University of California, San Francisco Dermatopathology Service, San Francisco, California

MELINDA R. MOHR, MD
Dermatology Resident, Department of Dermatology, Eastern Virginia Medical School, Norfolk, Virginia

MELISSA PECK PILIANG, MD
Departments of Dermatology and Anatomic Pathology, Cleveland Clinic, Cleveland Clinic Foundation, Cleveland, Ohio

PUSHKAR A. PHADKE, MD, PhD
Resident in Anatomic Pathology, Department of Pathology, Tufts Medical Center, Tufts University, Boston, Massachusetts

VICTOR G. PRIETO, MD, PhD
Departments of Pathology and Dermatology, University of Texas MD Anderson Cancer Center, Houston, Texas

GERALD S. SALDANHA, MBChB, PhD, FRCPath, MRCP
Senior Lecturer, Department of Cancer Studies and Molecular Medicine, Leicester Royal Infirmary, Leicester, United Kingdom

MARTIN J. TROTTER, MD, PhD, FRCPC
Associate Professor, Department of Pathology and Laboratory Medicine, University of Calgary, Calgary Laboratory Services, Calgary, Alberta, Canada

MAYA ZAYOUR, MD
Visiting Fellow, Yale Dermatopathology Laboratory, Department of Dermatology, Yale University School of Medicine, New Haven, Connecticut

DANIEL C. ZEDEK, MD
Clinical Instructor of Pathology and Dermatology, University of California, San Francisco, San Francisco, California

ARTUR ZEMBOWICZ, MD, PhD
Associate Professor, Department of Pathology, Tufts Medical Center, Tufts University, Boston, Massachusetts; Dermatopathologist, Lahey Clinic, Burlington, Massachusetts; Medical Director, www.DermatopathologyConsultations.com; Founder, www.Dermpedia.org

Contents

FORTHCOMING ISSUES

September 2011

Mass Spectrometry

Nigel Clarke, PhD,
Guest Editor

December 2011

Cytogenetics

Caroline Astbury, PhD, FACMG,
Guest Editor

RECENT ISSUES

March 2011

Veterinary Laboratory Medicine

Mary M. Christopher, DVM, PhD,
Guest Editor

December 2010

Genetics of Neurologic and Psychiatric Diseases

Alan Wells, MD, DMSc,
Guest Editor

September 2010

Prenatal Screening and Diagnosis

Anthony Odibo, MD, MSCE, and
David Krantz, MA,
Guest Editors

Preface

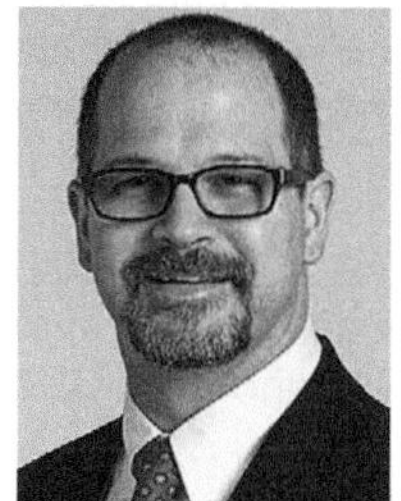

Steven D. Billings, MD
Guest Editor

Dermatopathology is an ever-changing field in the area of surgical pathology. Despite many advances, interpretation of melanocytic neoplasms remains a significant source of diagnostic difficulty encountered by surgical pathologists every day. "Is this lesion an unusual nevus?" and "Is this a subtle variant of melanoma?" are common dilemmas and questions faced on a daily basis.

In the selection of the articles for this issue, I hope to focus readers on especially problematic areas in the field of interpretation of melanocytic lesions. Interpretation of routine intradermal nevi and typical cases of superficial spreading melanoma do not pose significant difficulties, but a wide variety of melanocytic neoplasms do cause problems. In this issue, the topics have been selected to highlight melanocytic lesions that are a frequent source of diagnostic difficulty. These include a variety of benign melanocytic lesions, such as dysplastic nevi, congenital nevi, nevi of special anatomic sites, blue nevi and related entities, and Spitz nevi. The most diagnostically treacherous variants of melanoma, including spitzoid melanoma, desmoplastic melanoma, acral lentiginous melanoma, and nevoid melanoma, are also reviewed in detail. Each presentation provides a thorough review of these diagnostically challenging entities and emphasizes practical approaches to the diagnosis of these lesions.

In addition to a more traditional approach of focusing on histologic features of specific entities, I thought that it was important to also include articles dealing with practical day-to-day issues on specimen handling, specifically in relationship to melanoma. There is an article that provides an assessment on methods for handling specimens in order to more effectively evaluate surgical margins on melanoma cases. There is also an article that provides a guide to the handling and interpretation of sentinel lymph node biopsy specimens. Both of these articles provide practical guidance on these critical issues in managing melanoma cases.

The final article provides a glimpse into the future. Interpretation of melanocytic neoplasms will always be difficult. Insight into the molecular biology of melanocytic tumors is the new forefront that will provide new diagnostic tools for this endeavor. This article reviews current knowledge of the molecular biology of melanocytic neoplasms. This type of information will ultimately be the source of the development of new diagnostic tests and insights into the interpretation of melanocytic neoplasms.

Clin Lab Med 31 (2011) xi–xii
doi:10.1016/j.cll.2011.04.001
0272-2712/11/$ – see front matter

I know I learned a great deal reading the excellent information in this issue, and I am humbled by the opportunity to edit this text. The efforts of the contributing authors have resulted in an outstanding summary of and focus on difficult areas in interpretation of melanocytic neoplasms. I am confident that this issue will have a prominent place in many bookshelves in many offices, the Web site will have many and frequent visitors, and the material will be a valuable diagnostic aid.

Steven D. Billings, MD
Section of Dermatopathology, Anatomic Pathology
Cleveland Clinic, Cleveland, OH, USA

Department of Anatomic Pathology
Cleveland Clinic
9500 Euclid Avenue
L25, Cleveland, OH 44195, USA

E-mail address:
billins@ccf.org

Nevi of Special Sites

Ashley R. Mason, MD, Melinda R. Mohr, MD, Laine H. Koch, MD,
Antoinette F. Hood, MD*

KEYWORDS

- Nevi of special sites • Vulvar nevi • Flexural nevi
- Acral nevi • Ear nevi • Scalp nevi

OVERVIEW

Nevi of special sites (NOSS) encompass a class of benign nevi that show atypical histologic features akin to those of malignant melanomas or dysplastic nevi. NOSS may exist along a histologic spectrum of melanocytic lesions such as small melanocytic nevi (<5 mm), lentiginous nevi, dysplastic nevi, lentiginous melanoma, lentigo maligna, and nevi of special sites.[1] An expanding list of special sites includes the embryonic milkline/flexural sites, genitalia, acral sites, ear, and scalp (**Table 1**). NOSS may reflect regional diversity in skin structure and function. It is well known that skin microanatomy varies among sites in terms of epidermal thickness, appendage distribution, melanocyte distribution, dermal-epidermal junction structure, dermal structure, and blood supply.[2]

Although the etiology of NOSS remains conjectural, embryologic development may also partially explain the genesis of NOSS. Shared atypical features among milkline NOSS may imply a common ectodermal origin. Nevus cells are melanocytes and thus are derivatives of neural crest cells—pleuripotent derivatives of ectoderm.[3] The milklines arise from a bandlike thickening of ectoderm in the 4-week-old embryo and extend from the axillae to the inguinal folds.[4]

Some investigators[5] dispute the uniqueness of NOSS histologic features; however, the literature supports recognition of the patterns seen in this group of nevi. As NOSS often exhibit histologic features in common with melanoma, histopathologic criteria that define stereotypical benign nevi are not applicable to all skin sites. This article reviews in detail the histopathologic patterns seen in NOSS.

A version of this article was previously published in *Surgical Pathology Clinics* 2:3.
All coauthors deny conflicts of interests and have no financial disclosures.
Department of Dermatology, Eastern Virginia Medical School, 721 Fairfax Avenue, Suite 200, Norfolk, VA 23507, USA
* Corresponding author.
E-mail address: hoodaf_194110@evms.edu

Clin Lab Med 31 (2011) 229–242
doi:10.1016/j.cll.2011.03.001 labmed.theclinics.com

Key Features
Nevi of special sites (NOSS)

1. Special sites include the embryonic milkline/flexural sites, genitalia, palms, soles, ear, and scalp.
2. Not all nevi that occur in special sites are NOSS. At all special sites, stereotypical benign melanocytic nevi remain distinct diagnoses.
3. NOSS may have histologic features in common with melanoma.
4. NOSS nomenclature is not standardized. Other names for NOSS include: atypical genital nevi (AGN), atypical melanocytic nevus of the genital type (AMNGT), melanocytic acral nevus with intraepithelial ascent of cells (MANIACs), acral-lentiginous nevus of plantar skin, atypical nevi of the scalp, and special site nevi.
5. NOSS of flexural/milkline skin, genitalia, and scalp share similar histology—notably enlarged junctional nests with diminished cohesion of melanocytes.
6. Ear and breast NOSS are more atypical than nevi at other sites.
7. Scalp and acral NOSS have prominent pagetoid spread.
8. NOSS are thought to have a similar prognosis to stereotypical benign melanocytic nevi, but the long-term biologic behavior of NOSS is unknown.
9. Surgical excision with clear margins is recommended for all NOSS.

GROSS FEATURES

The gross appearance of NOSS varies among sites and has not been consistently described as unique from banal nevi occurring at special sites. Genital NOSS are often found in young women and represent approximately 5% of benign vulvar nevi.[6] Anecdotal reports claim that genital NOSS occur on the penis,[7] but their clinical appearance has not been described. Scrotal NOSS are categorized as a type of flexural nevi.[8] Flexural skin is defined as any curved part of the skin.[8]

Table 1
Nevi of special sites

Special Site	Locations
Genital nevi	• Vulva • Penis[7,a]
Flexural nevi	• Nevi of the milkline o Axillae o Breast o Inguinal folds • Other flexural sites o Umbilicus o Scrotum o Perianum
Acral nevi	• Ears • Palms • Soles • Knees[15,a] • Elbows[15,a]
Scalp	

[a] Anecdotal reports only.

Acral sites include the peripheral parts: the limbs, fingers, and ears.[9] Nevi on the palms and soles have linear striations corresponding to the dermatoglyphics of acral skin.[10] Scalp NOSS have primarily been identified in adolescents, and nevi may gradually darken or increase in size or elevation during adolescence.[11] **Table 2** summarizes the clinical features of histologically confirmed NOSS.

MICROSCOPIC FEATURES

Genital NOSS

Genital NOSS are characterized by the prominent, junctional proliferation of round-to-oval nests that may become confluent. Three architectural patterns have been described:

1. Nested pattern: large, often oval nests are oriented perpendicular or parallel to the dermal-epidermal junction (**Fig. 1**);
2. Dyshesive nest pattern: nearly contiguous dyshesive nests form a band that separates the epidermis from mature dermal melanocytes
3. Crowded pattern: ill-defined nests and single cells are closely apposed, obscuring the dermal-epidermal junction.[7]

Genital NOSS may also display the following concerning features: diffuse moderate to severe cytologic atypia, epithelioid cells with prominent nucleoli, focal central pagetoid spread (though rarely above the granular layer), and a broad zone of superficial

Table 2
Clinical appearance of nevi of special sites

Special Site		
Synonyms	**Location**	**Clinical Appearance of NOSS**
Genitalia • Atypical genital nevi (AGN)[6] • Atypical melanocytic nevus of the genital type (AMNGT)[7]	Unspecified	• Black (one-third)[7] • Brown (two-thirds)[7]
	Labia majora and perineum	• Elevated[7] • Mushroom-shaped[7]
	Labia minora and clitoris	• Macular[7]
Flexures	Milkline	• No data
Acral skin • Acral-lentiginous nevus of plantar skin[19] • Melanocytic acral nevus with intraepithelial ascent of cells (MANIACs)[15,26]	Soles	• Brown to dark brown macules[19] • Small (<10 mm)[19] • Uniform in color[19] • Regular borders[19]
	Palms	• No data
	Auricular region,[21] external auricule,[20] postauricular cheek,[20] and preauricular skin[20]	• Symmetric[21] • Ill-demarcated[21] • Approximately half are at least 6 mm[21]
Scalp • Atypical nevi of the scalp in adolescents[22]	Unspecified	• Dark brown • Clonal nevi ("fried-egg nevi"): light brown with darker raised center[11,32] • Rim nevi ("eclipse nevi"): flat, pink, or light brown with a darker brown peripheral rim[11,32]

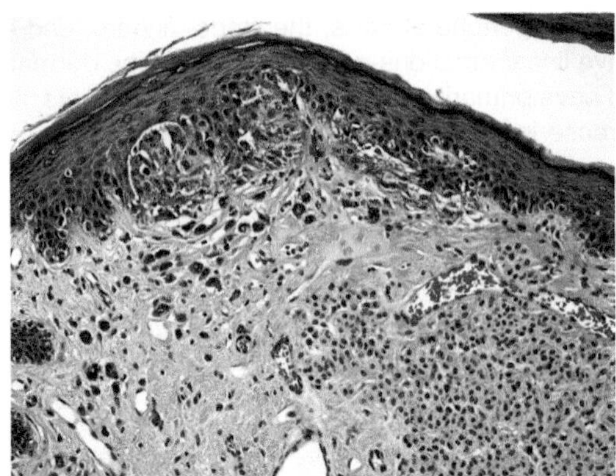

Fig. 1. Genital NOSS. A nested pattern of large, dyshesive nests oriented perpendicular to the dermal-epidermal junction is seen. Lentiginous proliferation and dermal fibroplasia are present (hematoxylin and eosin ×100).

dermal fibrosis.[6] In genital NOSS, an underlying population of benign-appearing, dermal nevus cells often forms a mushroom shape, and atypical nevus cells overlie the figurative mushroom cap (**Fig. 2**).[6,7] Reassuring features found in genital NOSS include symmetry, well-demarcated borders of the lesion, dermal maturation, and low dermal mitotic activity.[6]

Milkline/Flexural NOSS

A study of 40 flexural nevi showed that 22 were truly special site nevi with histologic features of genital NOSS.[8] Of these 22 nevi, most samples were from umbilicus (40%) and axillae (32%), and the remainder of the special site nevi were from the

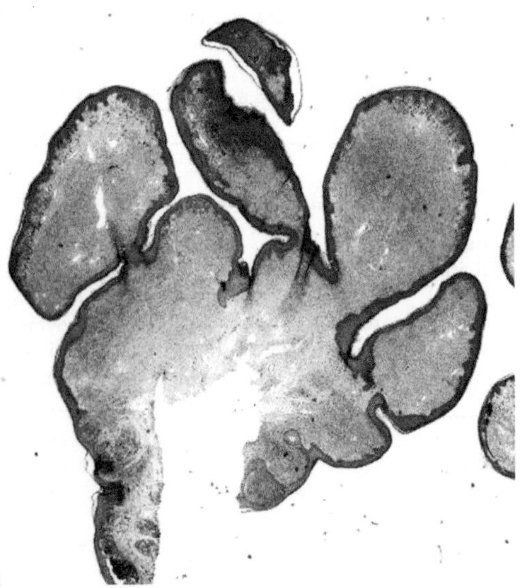

Fig. 2. Genital NOSS. Prominent mushroom-shaped morphology is evident at low magnification. Note the overall lesional symmetry (hematoxylin and eosin ×20).

inguinal creases, pubis, scrotum, and perianal skin.[8] Genital and flexural nevi histologically share the following features: fibroplasia in the papillary dermis, maturation, lentiginous melanocytic proliferation, and extension of intraepidermal component along adnexae.[8] Genital and flexural NOSS both manifest a "nested and dyshesive" pattern: enlarged junctional nests and diminished cohesion of melanocytes.[8] The characteristic large junctional nests of genital and flexural nevi vary in size, shape, and position.[8] In contrast to the moderate to severe atypia seen in genital NOSS, flexural NOSS nuclei are generally mildly to moderately atypical.[8] In the dermis, maturation of flexural NOSS cells and the absence of mitotic activity are notable.[8]

Breast NOSS histology has been studied separately from other milkline/flexural nevi. Breast NOSS often exhibit intraepidermal melanocytes above the basal layer, which occur singly or in groups, over an expanse of 3 rete ridges.[12] Breast NOSS also may display papillary dermal fibroplasia and melanocytic atypia (**Fig. 3**).[12]

Acral NOSS

Palmar/plantar NOSS may show upward migration of melanocytes.[10,13,14] The acronym MANIAC (Melanocytic Acral Nevus with Intraepithelial Ascent of Cells) describes these lesions (**Fig. 4**).[15] Retention of pigment may occur in the overlying stratum corneum, and may be physiologically related to the upwardly migrating cells. Nests can be large but usually show symmetry, and are often surrounded by a cleft so that nests appear well demarcated from adjacent keratinocytes.[10,13,16–18] Bridging between rete may be seen in up to 85% of benign acral nevi.[13,14]

The dermal component shows maturation, bland cytology, and lack of mitotic activity.[17] In addition, a bandlike inflammatory infiltrate may be present in acral nevi. This infiltrate is occasionally associated with fibroplasia or focal disappearance of the intraepidermal melanocytes.[19]

In a recent study, 42% of 101 junctional and compound nevi of the ear were identified as "unique" (ie, ear NOSS) whereas the remainder were banal nevi.[20] A subset of 69% of ear NOSS (26 nevi in total) showed uniformly large melanocytes, large vesicular nuclei without prominent nucleoli, and abundant pale, finely granular cytoplasm.[20] In a different study of 21 ear NOSS, approximately 50% cases were notable for moderate to severe cytologic atypia; however, the absence of mitotic figures and

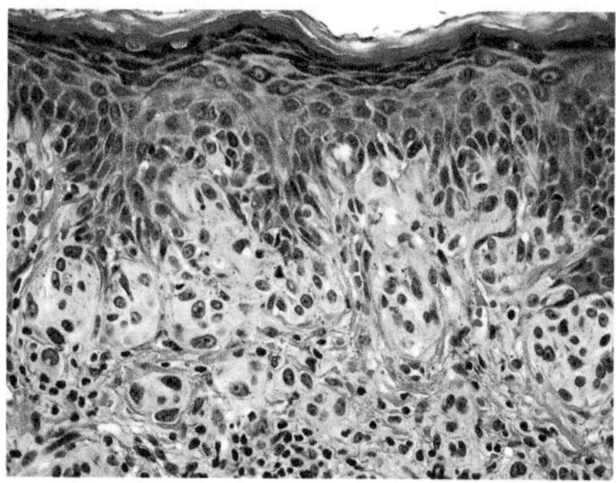

Fig. 3. Breast NOSS. Nuclear atypia is present but no specific pattern of nesting is seen (hematoxylin and eosin ×200).

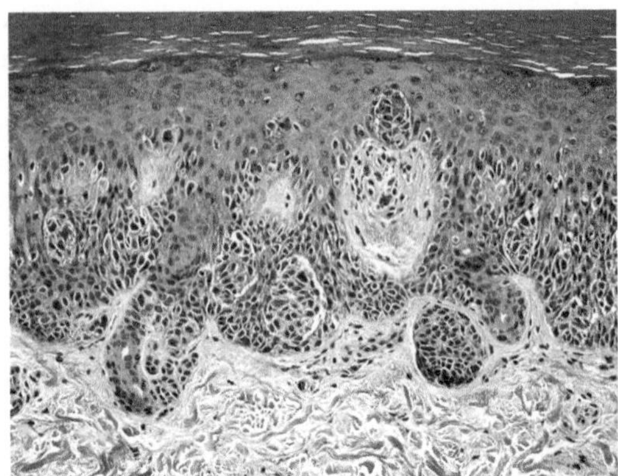

Fig. 4. Acral NOSS. Pagetoid spread of melanocytes in the epidermis is seen. The nests of melanocytes are irregular and confluent. The nests are located predominantly at the tips and shoulders of the rete ridges (hematoxylin and eosin $\times$100).

apoptotic melanocytes in all cases were reassuring as to the benign nature of these lesions.[21]

The most characteristic architectural feature of ear NOSS in one study was irregularity of the nesting pattern, in shape, size, and location, among the rete ridges.[20] Other characteristic features of the ear NOSS were poor circumscription, lateral extension of the junctional component beyond the dermal component, elongation of rete ridges, bridging between rete ridges, confluent nests of melanocytes, and dermal lymphocytic infiltrate.[20] Stromal reaction was observed in 81% of 21 ear NOSS in one study.[21] The majority of stromal reaction was a combination of lymphocytic infiltrate and dermal fibroplasia rather than dermal fibroplasia or lymphocytic infiltrate alone.[21]

Scalp NOSS

These nevi have been described histologically as poorly circumscribed and asymmetric.[22] Nests can be strikingly variable in size and shape and often become large.[22] Nests may also vary in location along the dermal-epidermal junction. The apparent random scattering of nests at the junction is characteristic, with rounder nests appearing at the base of the rete ridges.[22] Nests can be located not only at the base but also at the tip of the rete ridges. Nests may also extend into the follicular or adnexal units; some investigators[22] note that the most distinctive feature of scalp NOSS is the presence of large, bizarrely shaped nested melanocytes scattered along the junction within the follicle (**Fig. 5**). Melanocytic nests demonstrate lentiginous proliferation along the basal layer and may even demonstrate bridging among adjacent rete ridges.[22,23]

As with acral nevi, scalp nevi can demonstrate pagetoid spread of melanocytes above the dermal-epidermal junction.[13,17,22] Of note, this distinctive finding of upward or pagetoid spread has been seen in scalp nevi of adolescents but has not been observed in scalp nevi of adults or younger children.[22] This appearance may correlate grossly to that of the "fried-egg" nevi or "rim nevi" seen more frequently in adolescents.

Both lamellar and concentric fibroplasias have been described in the dermis, as well as the presence of mild to moderate inflammation.[23] This inflammatory infiltrate, if present, is typically mild and focal. Cytologic changes include an increase in the

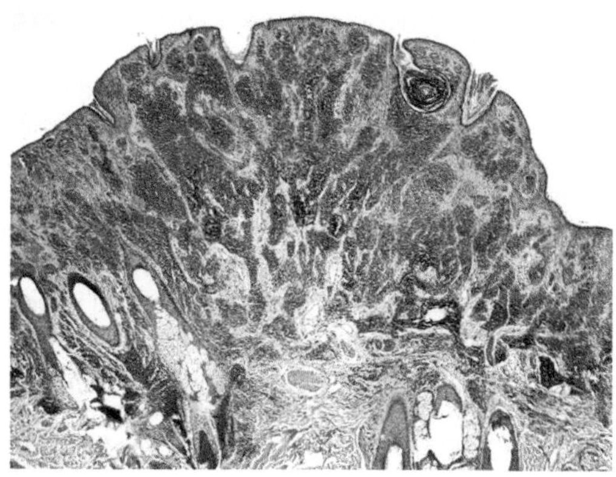

Fig. 5. Scalp NOSS. Large, bizarrely shaped nests of variable size and shape are evident at the dermal-epidermal junction with extension down follicular epithelium. Note also the absence of dermal fibroplasia or a significant lymphocytic infiltrate (hematoxylin and eosin ×40). (*Courtesy of* Robert J. Pariser, MD, Eastern Virginia Medical School, Norfolk, VA.)

size of nevoid cells as well as of large, hyperchromatic nuclei.[22,23] Cytologic atypia may be present but is usually mild to moderate in nature.[22,23]

DIFFERENTIAL DIAGNOSIS

The definitive diagnosis of NOSS is often ambiguous for 2 reasons: (1) special sites are not exempt from diagnoses of authentic dysplastic nevi or melanoma and (2) dysplastic nevi, melanoma, and NOSS share common histologic features. However, NOSS possess some distinctive, microscopic features.

Genital NOSS

Dysplastic nevi are characterized by a disorganized proliferation of single cells and small nests, rather than the larger dyshesive nests seen in genital NOSS.[6] The cytologic atypia of dysplastic nevi tends to be focal and random, in contrast to the relatively uniform atypia of genital NOSS. Also, in dysplastic nevi the pattern of dermal fibrosis tends to be concentric eosinophilic fibroplasia and lamellar fibroplasia, in contrast to the broad zone of dense fibrosis of the papillary and reticular dermis or no fibrosis in genital NOSS. Moreover, finely granular cytoplasmic melanin and

Differential Diagnosis
Nevi of special sites

- Stereotypical benign melanocytic nevi
- Dysplastic nevi
- Melanomas
- Congenital nevi
- Spitz nevi
- Traumatized nevi

Management of these melanocytic tumors is varied. Therefore, accurate diagnosis is essential.

perivascular infiltrate with pigment incontinence are seen more frequently in dysplastic nevi than in genital NOSS.[6]

Differentiation of a genital NOSS from superficial spreading or mucosal lentiginous melanoma can be challenging.[7] Melanoma is characterized histologically by an atypical single cell proliferation, in contrast to nests seen in genital NOSS; the pattern of pagetoid spread in melanoma involves all layers of the epidermis and is more widely distributed across the lesion.[6] Also, melanomas possess more severe cytologic atypia, dermal mitoses, and lack of dermal maturation and symmetry in comparison with genital NOSS.[6] Beyond histology, demographics are an important consideration in the diagnosis of vulvar melanoma, which typically affects postmenopausal women with a median age of 65 to 70 years.[7] One group advocates that the diagnosis of vulvar melanoma in someone younger than 40 years be made with caution.[7] In contrast, genital NOSS occur in young women with an average age of 21 years.[24]

Acral NOSS

Palmar/plantar NOSS may possess features similar to malignant melanoma such as the presence of upward migration, bridging of rete, an inflammatory infiltrate, and fibroplasia.[10,13–16] However, bridging between rete in acral nevi does not indicate increased risk for melanoma.[16] In fact, up to 85% of benign acral nevi can have bridging.[13,14] Upward migration seen in palmar/plantar NOSS also differs from that seen in melanoma in that the pagetoid infiltration of the epidermis occurs from small groups or nests of cells that lack atypia.[13,14,16] Pigment in the stratum corneum can be seen in both acral NOSS and melanoma.[16]

According to one study,[13] almost 40% of acral nevi have a significant inflammatory infiltrate, although the infiltrate is generally less than that seen in melanoma.[16] The infiltrate in acral NOSS is occasionally associated with fibroplasia or focal disappearance of the intraepidermal melanocytes.[19] In melanoma, the lymphocytic infiltrate tends to be patchy and, if regression is present, associated with absence of melanocytes in the epidermis.[25]

As expected of its acral location, the ear NOSS display most features of MANIACs.[15,26] The ear's designation as a special site is important given that the ear is one of the most common sites per unit area for melanoma, especially in men.[27] However, no age or sex predilection has been described for ear NOSS.[20]

Ear NOSS display elongation of rete ridges, continuous proliferation of melanocytes at the dermal-epidermal junction, and poor lateral circumscription characteristic of MANIACs; however, intraepidermal ascent is debatable. One study[21] found pagetoid spread in 12 of 21 (81%) ear NOSS cases, in contrast to a somewhat larger study[20] in which no melanocytes were observed above the dermal-epidermal junction in 42 cases. The pagetoid spread in ear NOSS involves single melanocytes, in contrast to pagetoid spread in melanoma characterized by clusters of 2 or more intraepidermal melanocytes.[21] Ear NOSS may share some histologic features with melanoma, including irregular nests at the dermal-epidermal junction, moderate to severe cytologic atypia, and pagetoid spread.[21] Thus, the distinction between ear NOSS and melanoma can be challenging.

Flexural NOSS

In comparison to stereotypical benign nevi, flexural NOSS display greater variability in the size of junctional nests as well as the location of nests at edges of rete and inter-rete—both features of dysplastic nevi.[8] Flexural NOSS and dysplastic nevi also show other similarities. Both display a tendency toward dermal fibroplasias and lentiginous melanocyte proliferation,[28] and, in addition, one-half of flexural NOSS have lateral extension and lymphocytic infiltrate characteristic of dysplastic nevi.[8] However, flexural NOSS lack cytologic atypia and lack associated stromal alterations seen commonly in dysplastic nevi.[28]

The differential diagnosis of a pigmented lesion on the breast includes benign melanocytic nevus, melanoma, pigmented mammary Paget disease, and pigmented epidermotropic metastatic breast carcinoma. Primary cutaneous melanoma of the breast is rare, accounting for less than 5% of all melanomas.[29] Pigmented mammary Paget disease and pigmented epidermotropic breast carcinoma may mimic melanoma both clinically and histologically; thus, immunohistochemistry is often necessary to confirm a diagnosis.[30] It is important to bear in mind that tumor cells of mammary Paget disease may express S100 protein. Therefore, melanocyte-specific markers in conjunction with epithelial markers should be considered in this differential diagnosis.

Scalp NOSS

Histologic criteria of poor circumscription and asymmetry were among the criteria used in the literature to call scalp nevi dysplastic.[22] However, if scalp nevi are likened to benign acral nevi, which demonstrate similar features, it can be said that these are not signs of dysplasia but rather distinct findings for these nevi of special sites.

DIAGNOSIS

As NOSS are inherently benign, accurate histopathologic diagnosis of NOSS translates into decreased reexcisions and surgical morbidity for the patient. Diagnostic acumen is especially important at cosmetically sensitive special sites such as the breast, genitalia, and scalp; however, the diagnosis of NOSS can be difficult given the lack of diagnostic criteria that are specific to NOSS. Currently, only small case series or small retrospective studies describe NOSS at each special site. Comparative studies of NOSS do not exist. **Table 3** summarizes key diagnostic features regarding nevi of each special site.

In a study of flexural NOSS, the investigators[12] make the following summary statements: (1) pagetoid spread is prominent in acral NOSS; (2) flexural and genital NOSS have enlarged junctional nests with diminished cohesion of melanocytes; and (3) breast NOSS have no specific pattern but are more atypical than nevi from other sites. In addition, new generalizations may be made: ear NOSS, like breast NOSS, are more atypical than nevi at other sites; scalp NOSS, like flexural and genital NOSS, have enlarged nests with discohesion of melanocytes[22]; and scalp NOSS, like acral nevi, have distinctive pagetoid spread albeit perhaps less frequently.[22]

Each melanocytic lesion with atypical features should be critically approached with full knowledge of the site of biopsy. Rigid application of histologic criteria for diagnosis of melanocytic lesions is counterproductive. Instead, the dermatopathologist must critically look at each lesion on a case-by-case and site-by-site basis, given the histologic nuances among NOSS.

PROGNOSIS

True NOSS are thought to have a benign course. In a series of 56 cases of genital NOSS, only one local recurrence was reported after incomplete excision, which was reexcised without further recurrence. No distant spread or metastasis has been reported for genital NOSS. No adequate follow-up was available in the study of 40 flexural NOSS.[20] Regarding breast nevi, the literature contains one reported case of primary cutaneous melanoma of the nipple, arising in a preexisting nevus present

Table 3
Histologic comparison among nevi of special sites

	Genitalia	Flexural Skin/Milkline		Acral Skin		Scalp (Adolescents)
	Vulva Penis[b]	Axillae, inguinal folds, umbilicus, scrotum, perianum, pubis	Breast	Ears	Palms & Soles	
Architectural pattern						
• Circumscription	Present[6]	ND	Present[12]	Minority[20,21]	Present[10,13,16,19]	Poor[22]
• Symmetry	Present[6]	ND	Present[12]	Present[20,21]	Present[10,13]	Asymmetric[22]
• Nests	• Diminished cohesion[6,7] • Varied size[6,7] • Often oval in shape[6,7] • 3 patterns: 1. Nested 2. Dyshesive 3. Crowded	• Diminished cohesion[8] • Varied size, shape, and position at dermal-epidermal junction[8] • Horizontal confluence of enlarged nests[8]	ND	• Irregular[20,21] • Confluent[20] • Located at rete tips & shoulders >> tips only[21]	• Large[19] • Variable size, shape[14,19] • Positioned at dermal-epidermal junction[14,19]	• Large, confluent[22] • Variable in shape[22] • Apparent random scattering[22] • Located at rete shoulders & tips[22]
• Lentiginous proliferation	Present[6]	Present[8]	Absent[12]	Present[20]	Present[14,16,19]	Present[22]
• Rete ridges	Bridging[6]	ND	ND	Elongated, bridging[20]	Elongated,[16,19] bridging[13]	ND

• Lateral extension	Present[6]	Present[8]	Absent[12]	Present[20]	Present[14,16,19]	ND
Melanocytes						
• Nuclear Atypia	Present (moderate to severe)[6]	Present (mostly mild to moderate)[8]	Present (not graded)[12]	Minority[20,a] versus majority (moderate to severe)[21]	Present (mild to moderate)[13,14,16]	Present[22]
• Mitoses	Rare dermal mitoses[6]	Absent[8]	ND	Absent	Rare[19]	ND
• Pagetoid spread	Present[6]	One case[8]	Present[12]	Absent[20,a] versus Present[21]	Present[10,13–16,19]	Minority[22]
• Maturation	Present[6]	Present[8]	Present[12]	Present[20]	Present[19]	ND
Stromal response						
• Fibroplasia	Present[6]	All cases[8]	Present[12]	Present[20,21]	Present[13,16,19]	Absent[22]
• Lymphocytic infiltrate	Minority[6,7]	Minority[8]	Absent[12]	Present[20,21]	Present[13,16,19]	Mild and focal[22]

Key: Present, majority cases (greater than one-half of cases); Minority, less than one-half of cases; Absent, no cases; ND, not described.

[a] Discrepancy: see text.

[b] Anecdotal.

Pitfalls
Nevi of special sites

! No clear diagnostic criteria exist for NOSS.

! The differential diagnosis between melanomas, NOSS, and dysplastic nevi can be difficult, especially as all share histologic features.

! Overdiagnosis of NOSS as melanomas or dysplastic nevi can increase surgical and psychological morbidity.

for 30 years.[31] Therefore, just as in nevi of other sites, one should clinically monitor nevi for changes in symmetry, border, color, and size.

Close monitoring of acral nevi is important, as malignant transformation to melanoma can occur. Melanomas arising from palmoplantar skin, either de novo or from existing nevi, have historically portended a poor prognosis[16] and thus acral NOSS should also be clinically respected. In a series of 42 cases of ear NOSS, only one local recurrence was reported after incomplete excision; however, this case in addition to 40% of the other patients studied in this series were lost to follow-up.[20] The long-term sequelae of scalp NOSS is unknown.

Appropriate diagnosis of NOSS is important to avoid overdiagnosis of melanoma or dysplastic nevi and associated surgery, potential disfigurement, and patient concern. While more systematic studies of NOSS are awaited, removal of any concerning clinical lesion and conservative reexcision to obtain clear margins of NOSS is recommended. Close clinical follow-up is also prudent, as the true biologic potential of NOSS is not fully understood.

ACKNOWLEDGMENTS

Special thanks are extended to Drs John C. Maize Sr and John C. Maize Jr for their inspiration to further research nevi of special sites. Also, the authors would like to acknowledge Robert J. Pariser, MD for his editorial guidance and contribution of the scalp slide.

REFERENCES

1. Rabkin MS. The limited specificity of histological examination in the diagnosis of dysplastic nevi. J Cutan Pathol 2008;35(Suppl 2):20–3.
2. McGrath J, Eady R, Pope F. Anatomy and organization of human skin. In: Burns T, Breathnach S, Cox N, et al, editors, Rook's textbook of dermatology, vol. 1. 7th edition. Wiley-Blackwell; 2004. p. 3.1–3.84.
3. Gilbert SF. Developmental biology. 8th edition. Sunderland (MA): Sinauer Associates, Inc Publishers; 2006.
4. Sinnatamby CS, Last RJ. Last's anatomy: regional and applied. 11th edition. New York: Elsevier Health Sciences; 2006.
5. Urso C, Rongioletti F, Innocenzi D, et al. Histological features used in the diagnosis of melanoma are frequently found in benign melanocytic naevi. J Clin Pathol 2005;58(4):409–12.
6. Gleason BC, Hirsch MS, Nucci MR, et al. Atypical genital nevi. A clinicopathologic analysis of 56 cases. Am J Surg Pathol 2008;32(1):51–7.

7. Clark WH Jr, Hood AF, Tucker MA, et al. Atypical melanocytic nevi of the genital type with a discussion of reciprocal parenchymal-stromal interactions in the biology of neoplasia. Hum Pathol 1998;29(1 Suppl 1):S1–24.
8. Rongioletti F, Ball RA, Marcus R, et al. Histopathological features of flexural melanocytic nevi: a study of 40 cases. J Cutan Pathol 2000;27(5):215–7.
9. Stedman TL, Dirckx JH. Stedman's concise medical dictionary for the health professions. 4th edition. Philadelphia: Lippincott Williams & Wilkins; 2001.
10. Signoretti S, Annessi G, Puddu P, et al. Melanocytic nevi of palms and soles: a histological study according to the plane of section. Am J Surg Pathol 1999; 23(3):283–7.
11. Huynh PM, Glusac EJ, Bolognia JL. The clinical appearance of clonal nevi (inverted type A nevi). Int J Dermatol 2004;43(12):882–5.
12. Rongioletti F, Urso C, Batolo D, et al. Melanocytic nevi of the breast: a histologic case-control study. J Cutan Pathol 2004;31(2):137–40.
13. Boyd AS, Rapini RP. Acral melanocytic neoplasms: a histologic analysis of 158 lesions. J Am Acad Dermatol 1994;31(5 Pt 1):740–5.
14. Evans MJ, Gray ES, Blessing K. Histopathological features of acral melanocytic nevi in children: study of 21 cases. Pediatr Dev Pathol 1998;1(5):388–92.
15. LeBoit PE. A diagnosis for maniacs. Am J Dermatopathol 2000;22(6):556–8.
16. Fallowfield ME, Collina G, Cook MG. Melanocytic lesions of the palm and sole. Histopathology 1994;24(5):463–7.
17. Hosler GA, Moresi JM, Barrett TL. Nevi with site-related atypia: a review of melanocytic nevi with atypical histologic features based on anatomic site. J Cutan Pathol 2008;35(10):889–98.
18. Miyazaki A, Saida T, Koga H, et al. Anatomical and histopathological correlates of the dermoscopic patterns seen in melanocytic nevi on the sole: a retrospective study. J Am Acad Dermatol 2005;53(2):230–6.
19. Clemente C, Zurrida S, Bartoli C, et al. Acral-lentiginous naevus of plantar skin. Histopathology 1995;27(6):549–55.
20. Lazova R, Lester B, Glusac EJ, et al. The characteristic histopathologic features of nevi on and around the ear. J Cutan Pathol 2005;32(1):40–4.
21. Saad AG, Patel S, Mutasim DF. Melanocytic nevi of the auricular region: histologic characteristics and diagnostic difficulties. Am J Dermatopathol 2005;27(2):111–5.
22. Fabrizi G, Pagliarello C, Parente P, et al. Atypical nevi of the scalp in adolescents. J Cutan Pathol 2007;34(5):365–9.
23. Fernandez M, Raimer SS, Sanchez RL. Dysplastic nevi of the scalp and forehead in children. Pediatr Dermatol 2001;18(1):5–8.
24. Ribe A. Melanocytic lesions of the genital area with attention given to atypical genital nevi. J Cutan Pathol 2008;35(Suppl 2):24–7.
25. Ackerman A, Cerroni L, Kerl H. Pitfalls in histopathologic diagnosis of malignant melanoma. Philadelphia: Lea & Febiger; 1994. p. 147–82.
26. McCalmont TH, Brinsko R, LeBoit PE. Melanocytic acral nevi with intraepidermal ascent of cells (MANIACs): a reappraisal of melanocytic lesions from acral sties. Am J Dermatopathol 1991;18(1):378.
27. Elder DE. Skin cancer. Melanoma and other specific nonmelanoma skin cancers. Cancer 1995;75(Suppl 1):245–56.
28. Elder DE. Precursors to melanoma and their mimics: nevi of special sites. Mod Pathol 2006;19(Suppl 2):S4–20.
29. Kurul S, Tas F, Buyukbabani N, et al. Different manifestations of malignant melanoma in the breast: a report of 12 cases and a review of the literature. Jpn J Clin Oncol 2005;35(4):202–6.

30. Requena L, Sangueza M, Sangueza OP, et al. Pigmented mammary Paget disease and pigmented epidermotropic metastases from breast carcinoma. Am J Dermatopathol 2002;24(3):189–98.
31. Kinoshita S, Yoshimoto K, Kyoda S, et al. Malignant melanoma originating on the female nipple: a case report. Breast Cancer 2007;14(1):105–8.
32. Suh KY, Bolognia JL. Signature nevi. J Am Acad Dermatol 2009;60(3):508–14.

Nevoid Melanoma

A. Hafeez Diwan, MD, PhD[a,b,c,*], Alexander J. Lazar, MD, PhD[c,d]

KEYWORDS

- Nevoid melanoma • Diagnostic pitfalls • Deceptive histology
- Mitotic figures • Small cell melanoma • Nuclear atypia
- Immunohistochemical findings

Nevoid melanoma is the name given to a morphological subtype of melanoma. In 1980, Levene described it as a "pseudonevoid and verrucous melanoma."[1] The same histologic features have also been described by Blessing and colleagues[2] who studied 20 such cases in 1995, representing 3.2% of melanomas diagnosed at Aberdeen University in a period lasting from 1970 to 1991. It has been included in the type of melanoma referred to as "minimal deviation melanoma." The term minimal deviation expresses a feature that is central to the histology of nevoid melanoma: histologic features that are only slightly different from those of nevi, ie, features that are minimally deviated from what is acceptable in a nevus, but sufficiently distinct to allow recognition of its malignant nature.

It should be emphasized that "Spitzoid" melanomas, ie, melanomas that have features resembling Spitz nevus are not included by most authors in the term nevoid melanoma (although from a purely semantic viewpoint, melanomas that resemble Spitz nevi, could certainly be regarded as nevoid melanoma; in fact, Wong and colleagues[3] studied seven cases of nevoid melanomas that included spindled and epithelioid nevi as well as banal dermal nevi). Spitzoid melanomas are discussed in, the article by Zedek and colleagues elsewhere in this issue. Another descriptive term for nevoid melanoma is small-cell melanoma, as nevus cells are "small," and a melanoma that tends toward "smallness" gives rise to this histological appearance, similar to a nevus. Thus Kossard and Wilkinson used this term synonymously with nevoid melanoma.[4] Other authors do not share this view.[5] The key point in our opinion is that, however it is named, it should not be mistaken for a nevus.

It should be emphasized that nevoid melanoma refers to a particular deceptive histology. The term nevoid melanoma (or "minimal deviation" melanoma) should not

---

A version of this article was previously published in *Surgical Pathology Clinics* 2:3.

[a] Department of Pathology, Baylor College of Medicine, One Baylor Plaza, Suite 214B, MS: BCM 315, Houston, TX, USA
[b] Department of Dermatology, Baylor College of Medicine, Houston, TX, USA
[c] Department of Pathology, University of Texas MD Anderson Cancer Center, 1515 Holcombe, Unit 85, Houston, TX, USA
[d] Department of Dermatology, Sarcoma Research Center, The University of Texas MD Anderson Cancer Center, Houston, TX, USA
* Corresponding author.
E-mail address: ahdiwan@bmc.edu

Clin Lab Med 31 (2011) 243–253
doi:10.1016/j.cll.2011.03.002 **labmed.theclinics.com**

Key Features
Nevoid melanoma

1. Melanoma characterized by predominantly nevoid-appearing tumor cells.
2. The silhouette of the lesion at low power can be rather symmetrical and not overtly suspicious for melanoma.
3. Although the cells are nevoid, there is pleomorphism (albeit slight), and nuclear atypia; prominent nucleoli may be evident. This requires examination at higher power.
4. The junctional component may contain melanoma in situ, which is a good clue to the diagnosis.
5. Mitoses must be sought and can be found in the deeper portions of the lesion.
6. There is apparent maturation, but high-power examination often reveals that the nuclear size is not appreciably different in the lower parts of the lesion.
7. Nevoid melanoma can be difficult to define, in contrast to other types of melanoma. An unfortunate functional definition (ex post facto) is "a melanocytic neoplasm called a nevus, but with subsequent diagnostic regret."

be taken to imply that this form of melanoma has a more favorable clinical outcome. Schmoeckel and colleagues[6] and Zembowicz and colleagues[7] demonstrated that nevoid melanomas are not less aggressive than conventional melanomas, with prognosis guided by Breslow thickness as with all other forms of melanoma. For this reason, the microscopic assessment of traditional prognostic variables and the subsequent clinical staging of nevoid melanoma are no different than that of other melanomas. The importance of nevoid melanoma lies in that it can be a source of adverse consequences to the patient and to the pathologist who may miss the diagnosis. As nevoid melanoma can be so readily confused for a nevus, there may be a delay in diagnosis, allowing melanoma to progress to a higher stage before it is detected. Subsequent evaluation of prior pathology in a patient with, for example, Stage IV melanoma may uncover this diagnosis. But by this stage it is too late to positively impact patient outcome and the matter can become a medicolegal issue. This scenario, although uncommon, is not rare, and it has to be kept in mind so that diligent evaluation of any nevus that appears "different" or "funny-looking" is undertaken.

GROSS FEATURES

Clinically, nevoid melanomas present as papules, nodules, or verrucous lesions. They are black or brown, and may have a variegated appearance. Like nodular melanomas, the border may be smooth. Some dermatopathologists consider any melanoma including those with radial growth phase that have nevoid cells in the dermis as a nevoid melanoma. Both Schmoeckel and colleagues[6] and Blessing and colleagues[2] included nevoid melanomas with radial growth phase in their studies. In nevoid melanomas that have an intraepidermal, radial growth phase, the border may be irregular.

On cut surface, the lesion may be amelanotic and pink or may appear brown to black, extending to a variable distance below the epidermis and depending on the degree and distribution of pigmentation.

MICROSCOPIC FEATURES

The overlying epidermis may be relatively normal, acanthotic, verrucous, or somewhat attenuated (**Figs. 1–3**). There may or may not be an intraepidermal component

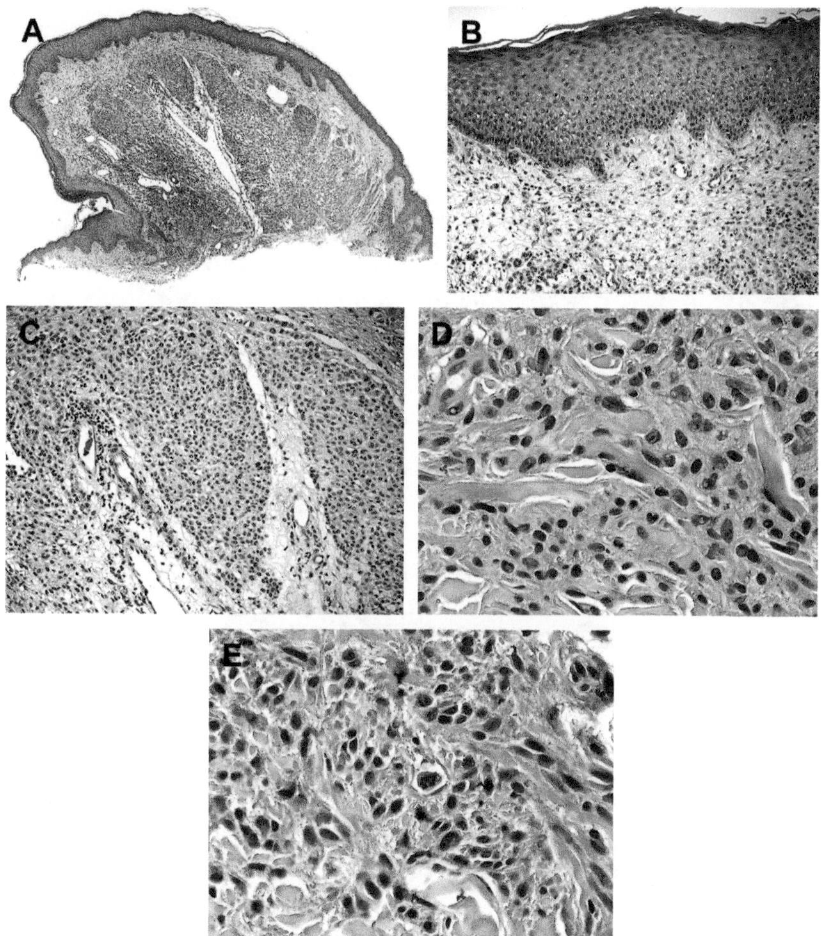

Fig. 1. (*A*) Scanning power H&E, showing deceptively nevic silhouette. (*B*) A ×200 H&E image, showing no epidermal component, and nevoid cells in upper dermis. (*C*) A ×200 H&E image showing crowded nevoid cells. (*D*) A ×400 H&E image showing cellular atypia and scattered nucleoli in the lower part of lesion. (*E*) A ×400 H&E image showing mitosis in lower portion of lesion.

(ie, melanoma in situ) composed of atypical, confluent, single, and nested melanocytes with pagetoid spread (**Figs. 4–6**). As mentioned previously, many consider nevoid melanoma as a subtype of nodular melanoma. Others may include under this term those with nevoid dermal cells but with a radial growth phase with extension of melanoma in situ beyond the boundaries intradermal component (by convention, for this to be classified as radial growth phase, this extension has to be more than three rete ridges away from the edge of the dermal component). Ulceration may be present (see **Fig. 6**), and when observed, is a good clue to the diagnosis and portends a higher stage (as with melanoma in general).

The intradermal component is, as the name suggests, rather nevoid in appearance (**Figs. 1–7**). At low power there is the appearance of maturation (see **Figs. 3** and **4**), both architecturally where nests decrease in size with depth to single cells and small

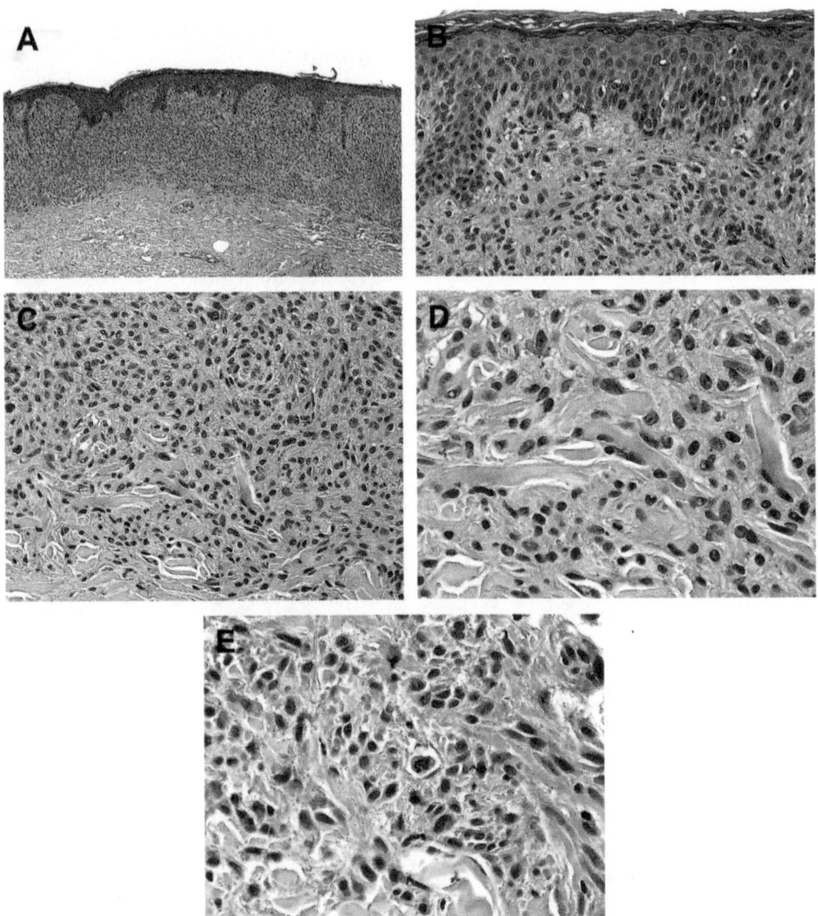

Fig. 2. (*A*) Scanning power H&E, showing nevoid architecture. (*B*) A ×200 H&E image showing epidermal component and plump nevoid cells (nucleoli are evident at this power). (*C*) A ×200 H&E image showing lower half of lesion with similar morphology. (*D*) A ×400 H&E image highlighting nucleoli. (*E*) A ×400 H&E image showing mitoses and scattered nucleoli.

clusters at the base and cytologically with the cells appearing small and relatively bland. Examination at higher power dispels the appearance of maturation. Invariably there is evidence of at least slight nuclear atypia with slight pleomorphism, hyperchromasia, irregular nuclear contours, and evident nucleoli (see **Figs. 1, 2** and **4**).[8] It may appear that the cells become progressively smaller with descent in the dermis, but close inspection demonstrates that the nuclei are roughly the same size at the top and bottom of the lesion. This unusual discordance between cellular and architectural maturation is a clue to this diagnosis. Nevertheless, many nevoid melanomas may truly show decreases in both overall and nuclear sizes; however, nuclear atypia, nucleoli, and hyperchromasia are still seen in the "mature" component (see **Figs. 4, 6** and **7**). Fine dusty melanin may be seen in some cases, again both in the top and bottom portions of the tumor (but it should be emphasized that this feature is not

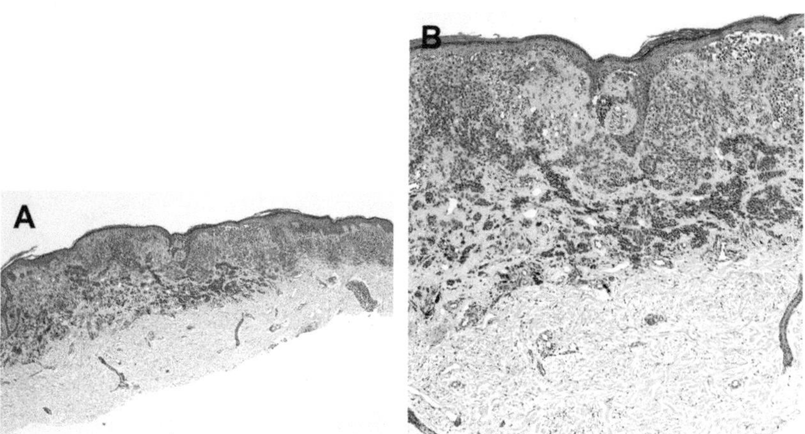

Fig. 3. (*A*) Scanning power H&E, showing nevoid appearance and apparent maturation. (*B*) A ×40 H&E image, showing apparent maturation.

invariable). Finally, mitotic figures, including atypical ones, may be found throughout the lesion. Spotting mitoses may initially require a diligent search.

IMMUNOHISTOCHEMISTRY

Immunohistochemical studies, when used in conjunction with a suspicious histology, can be useful in arriving at a diagnosis.[9]

HMB45, the antibody to melanosomal gp100, shows a characteristic pattern in nevi. The epidermal and possibly the upper dermal component show labeling with HMB45. However, the mid and lower dermal sections show reduced to absent labeling. In other words, there is progressive loss of HMB45 immunoreactivity with progressive descent in the dermis (see **Fig. 6**). This phenomenon is referred to maturation. Loss of maturation may be evidenced not just by reduced HMB45 immunoreactivity from top to bottom, but by irregular labeling (with patchy "hot-spots" of positivity), which does not follow an orderly decrease with descent in the dermis (see later in this article). Mib1, which is an antibody to Ki-67, is a surrogate marker for proliferation. Nevi are expected to have a low proliferation rate, unlike melanoma (see **Figs. 6** and **7**).

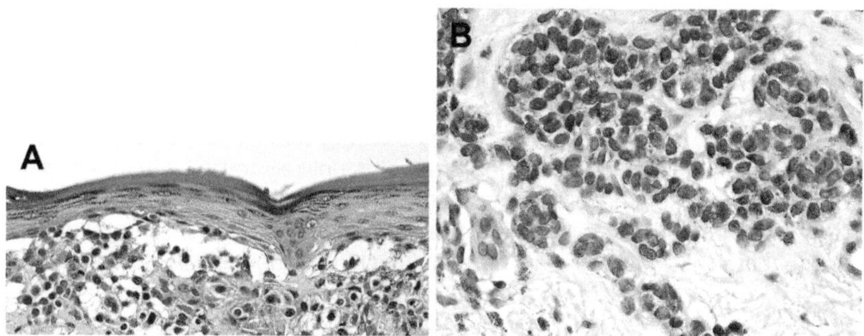

Fig. 4. Same lesion as in **Fig. 3** (*A*) A ×200 H&E image showing conspicuous melanoma in situ and more epithelioid dermal cells, indicative of invasive melanoma. (*B*) A ×400 H&E image showing lower portion, with apparently smaller cells.

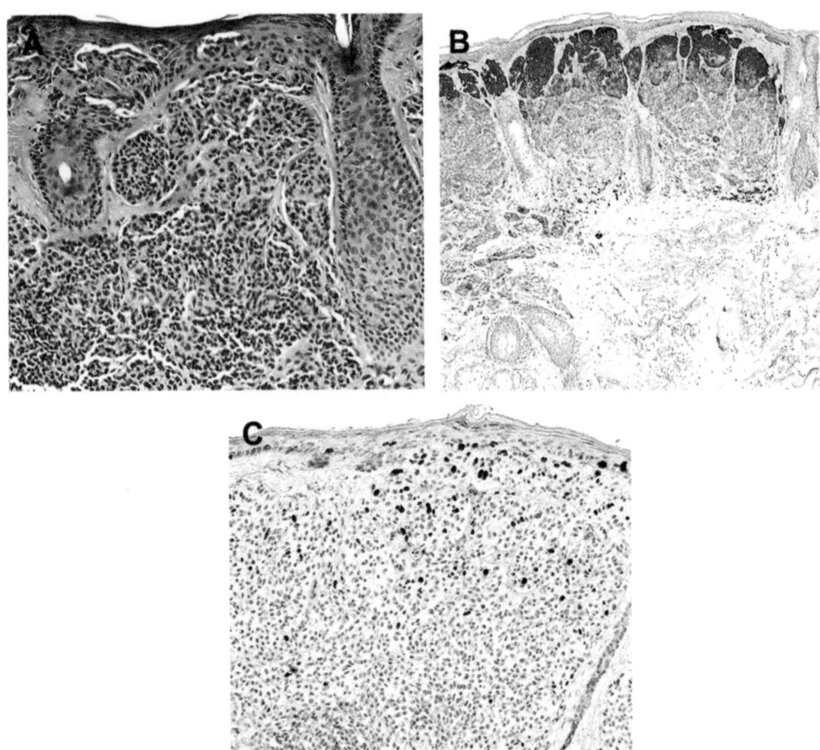

Fig. 5. (*A*) Nevoid melanoma with crowded, nevoid cells (×100, H&E). (*B*) HMB45 labeling (scanning magnification), showing loss of maturation with spotty labeling at the bottom of the lesion. (*C*) Ki-67 labeling (using Mib1 antibody) (×100) showing increased immunoreactivity. There is some maturation with decreased labeling in the lower part, but the overall labeling index is increased.

Different authors have proposed figures ranging from 6% to 20% labeling of nuclei with the Mib1 antibody as a marker for melanoma. As infiltrating lymphocytes often show Mib1 reactivity, double labeling with a melanocytic stain can be helpful to ensure that the Mib1 reactivity is actually in a melanocyte (see **Fig. 7**).

Mib1 labeling also shows maturation, similar to HMB45, in nevi, but not in melanoma. As with mitotic activity, Mib1 reactivity toward the base of the lesion is particularly a matter of concern. Thus an additional feature should be included in evaluating the results of these immunohistochemical studies: Irregular immunoreactivity with either of these two antibodies, with patchy staining that does not conform to any orderly pattern, is a very suspicious feature that is unlikely to be seen in nevus.

Multiple other markers have been studied that may have a role in the evaluation of nevoid melanoma.[10] These include cyclins A and B, cyclin D1/D3, metallothionein, p16, WT-1, and antibody to leptin receptor. Only rare nevi show greater than 5% labeling of cyclins A and B, as compared with greater than half of melanomas. Cyclin D1 immunopositivity is very infrequent in nevi as compared with melanoma; Spitz nevi, in addition, show maturation with this marker. p16 is seen more commonly in nevi than in melanoma (but expression in melanoma is nonetheless seen, albeit in fewer instances). WT-1 is not seen in benign nevi, but may be seen in a minority of dysplastic

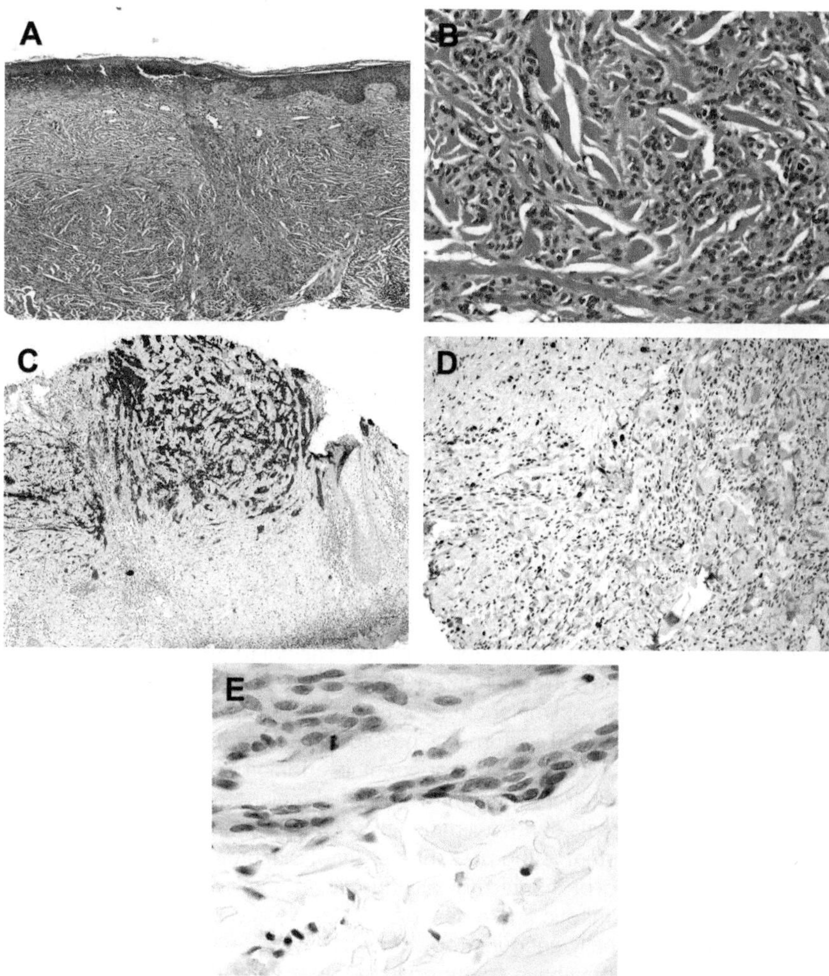

Fig. 6. Nevoid melanoma with ulceration. (*A*) Scanning magnification H&E showing nevoid cells in dermis, without an epidermal component. (*B*) A ×100 H&E image showing plump nevoid cells in the lower dermis. (*C*) HMB45 labels the entire lesion, showing lack of maturation. (*D*) Increased labeling for Ki-67 in the lower portion of lesion. (*E*) Negative control immunohistochemical slide showing mitosis in the base of the lesion.

nevi, and is frequently seen in Spitz nevi and melanoma. Metallothionein shows a maturation pattern in nevi but not in melanoma. Antileptin-receptor antibody labels nevi very poorly at best. When nevi do show immunoreactivity, they exhibit maturation. In contrast, melanoma shows diffuse leptin-receptor immunoreactivity, although this has not been specifically tested in a significant series of nevoid melanoma.[11] Many immunohistochemical markers have been purported to be helpful in the diagnosis of melanoma and distinguishing it from banal nevus. Often such markers are user dependent and require specific experience and reasoned judgment to be helpful in any particular situation. In our experience, the Ki-67 index, often supplemented with HMB-45, is the most useful in routine practice. Other immunohistochemical stains are often best used as a panel and an immunohistochemical result should never

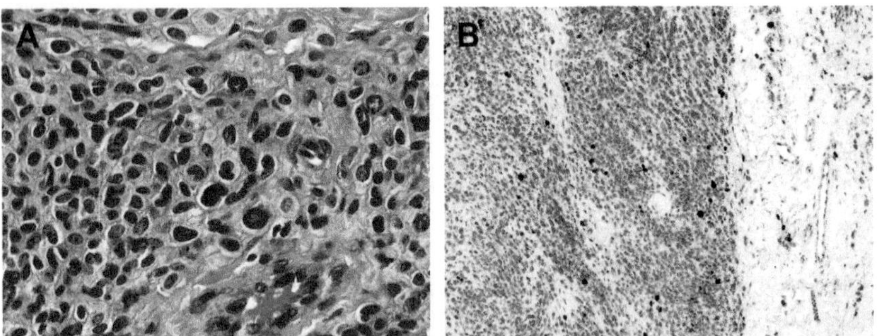

Fig. 7. (*A*) Nevoid appearing cells (H&E magnification ×200). (*B*) A double-labeled slide with anti-Mart1 decorating the cytoplasm and anti-Ki-67 labeling nuclei (×100). The proliferation rate is increased. (*Courtesy of* Dr Victor G. Prieto, The University of Texas MD Anderson Cancer Center.)

overrule a sound histologic assessment, but rather be used to gather evidence to support one's morphologic impression.

DIFFERENTIAL DIAGNOSIS

A few pertinent differentials must be kept in mind so as not to overdiagnose this entity. The presence of melanoma in situ in the overlying epidermis is not de facto proof of a diagnosis of invasive nevoid melanoma. Sometimes the dermal component is simply a nevus, and absence of the features of nevoid melanoma should lead one to the correct diagnosis. Also, if the dermal component, in addition to appearing like a nevus, is morphologically dissimilar from the intraepidermal melanoma, then there is greater reason to doubt a diagnosis of nevoid melanoma. Of all the features listed previously, perhaps the most important is the presence of mitotic figures (and/or elevated Mib1 reactivity), which should be hunted for assiduously in the dermis. The presence of even a single observed mitotic figure deep in the dermis is very concerning, although in practice more are usually encountered with scrutiny of the sections.

Congenital nevi, too, may have scattered intraepidermal melanocytic atypia, which should not be overinterpreted as melanoma in situ, leading one to misdiagnose the

Differential Diagnosis
Nevoid melanoma

1. Nevus
2. Melanoma in situ arising in association with a nevus: This is a differential for nevoid melanoma that has an intraepidermal component.
3. Congenital nevus: Congenital nevi may have atypical intraepidermal component, which may be mistaken for melanoma in situ; again, this is a differential for nevoid melanoma that has an intraepidermal component.
4. "Dysplastic" nevus
5. Combined nevus: with a blue nevus component
6. Inverted type A nevus
7. Keratotic nevus

entire nevus as a nevoid melanoma. A variation on this theme is melanoma in situ arising in a preexisting congenital nevus. As noted, this does not necessarily mean that the intradermal nevus is nevoid melanoma. The cytologic features should be present for a diagnosis of nevoid melanoma to be made. As always, immunohistochemical studies may be of great help in assisting the diagnostic process.

Because many nevoid melanomas may have a warty epidermis, a keratotic nevus or neoplasm is another differential (often more on the clinical impression), but may be easily distinguished from melanoma.

Nevoid melanomas may lack real maturation and two other differential diagnostic considerations should be mentioned. Combined nevus, for example an intradermal and cellular blue nevus, may show apparent lack of maturation, with larger, pigmented melanocytes of the blue nevus component at the base of the lesion. This should not be interpreted as nevoid melanoma. An HMB45 study can highlight the blue nevus component, with the remainder of the nevus exhibiting maturation. An inverted type A or clonal nevus contains the larger type A nevus cells at the base of the lesion. However, mitotic figures, nuclear atypia, and large nucleoli will not be evident, enabling distinction to be made.

Finally, metastatic melanoma, especially metastatic nevoid melanoma, may be the diagnosis when there is a minimal epidermal component, or if any epidermal component does not extend too far beyond the dermal melanoma. But these features may also be seen in nevoid melanoma and so the clinical context, including whether the patient has had a prior melanoma, and whether there are multiple, likely satellite lesions, are pointers to the correct diagnosis.

DIAGNOSIS

Biopsy diagnosis of nevoid melanoma is more challenging than the usual melanomas unless close attention is paid. Nevoid melanomas exhibit varying degrees of atypia present, and the more atypical ones are obviously easier to diagnose. Regardless, a low-power diagnosis is not sufficient and should be actively discouraged. Any pigmented or melanocytic lesion should be evaluated on at least medium power to highlight the atypical nuclear features including the nucleoli, mitoses (especially in the lower parts of the lesion), and the presence of pigment (also in the lower part of the lesion). The only features that may be easily observed at low power are (1) the closely packed cells or the increased cellularity, and (2) ulceration. Any "nevus" that appears too cellular, or has ulceration, should be viewed with the greatest suspicion and should be submitted to a detailed examination to look for the other findings listed previously.

PROGNOSIS

Nevoid melanoma is, as has been mentioned earlier, not a common diagnosis. There are no studies showing how frequent it is. However, there is no reason to suppose at this time that it represents any more than a morphologic subtype without any special prognostic significance. The same American Joint Committee on Cancer (AJCC) staging criteria apply to nevoid melanoma as for melanoma in general (with Stage I having an excellent prognosis, around 95% 5-year survival and Stage IV, a dismal prognosis, with median survival of 6 to 9 months). Depth of invasion (Breslow thickness) remains the most crucial determinant of prognosis. The presence of ulceration is a negative prognostic factor and increases the stage of the melanoma.

Even so, because there is a chance for a nevoid melanoma to be missed, it is possible that this delay in diagnosis assumes importance in determining overall

Pitfalls
Nevoid melanoma

! This morphological subtype of melanoma is easily mistaken for a nevus. The diagnosis may therefore be easily missed, with adverse medicolegal consequences.

! A nevus that appears too cellular or crowded should be evaluated at higher power to make sure that mitoses, pleomorphism, atypia, and pseudomaturation are not also present, these features being those of nevoid melanoma.

prognosis, with cases coming to light once the disease has advanced beyond the early stages of disease. Perhaps because nevoid melanoma is all too often a diagnosis made in retrospect after the lesion has been previously treated as a banal nevus, local recurrence and metastatic rates are reported at up to 50% with subsequent mortality of at least 25%.[7]

TREATMENT

The treatment of nevoid melanoma is no different than that of melanoma in general, with the exception that there is no in-situ nevoid melanoma (as nevoid melanoma, by definition, implies a nevoid dermal component). Thin melanomas (<1.0 mm) are best treated with a 1-cm margin; melanomas that are between 1 and 4 mm require a 2-cm margin, and for those thicker than 4 mm 2- to 3-cm margins are recommended. The requirements for sentinel node biopsy, lymph node dissection, and adjuvant therapy are the same as for melanoma in general. (At the University of Texas MD Anderson Cancer Center, we perform a sentinel node biopsy for melanomas that have any of the following features: ulceration, thickness >1.0 mm, the presence of vertical growth phase, Clark level IV, or extensive regression, but this approach is not universal at all centers.) Unfortunately, Stage IV melanoma, despite most treatment measures, carries a grave prognosis.

REFERENCES

1. Levene A. On the histological diagnosis and prognosis of malignant melanoma. J Clin Pathol 1980;33:101–24.
2. Blessing K, Evans AT, Al-Nafussi A. Verrucous nevoid and keratotic malignant melanoma: a clinico-pathologic study of 20 cases. Histopathology 1995;23: 453–8.
3. Wong TY, Suster S, Duncan LM, et al. Nevoid melanoma: a Clinicopathologic study of seven cases of malignant melanoma mimicking spindle and epithelioid cell nevus and verrucous dermal nevus. Hum Pathol 1995;26:171–9.
4. Kossard S, Wilkinson B. Nucleolar organizer regions and image analysis nuclear morphometry of small cell (nevoid) melanoma. J Cutan Pathol 1995;22:132–6.
5. Barnhill RL, Flotte TJ, Fleischli M, et al. Cutaneous melanoma and atypical Spitz tumors in childhood. Cancer 1995;76:1833–45.
6. Schmoeckel C, Castro CE, Braun-Falco O. Nevoid malignant melanoma. Arch Dermatol Res 1985;277:362–9.
7. Zembowicz A, McCusker M, Chiarelli C, et al. Morphological analysis of nevoid melanoma. A study of 20 cases with a review of the literature. Am J Dermatopathol 2001;23:167–75.
8. Massi G. Melanocytic nevi stimulant of melanoma with medicolegal significance. Virchows Arch 2007;451:623–47.

9. McNutt NS, Urmacher C, Hakimian J, et al. Nevoid malignant melanoma: morphologic patterns and immunohistochemical reactivity. J Cutan Pathol 1995;22: 502–17.
10. Carlson JA, Ross JS, Slominski AJ. New techniques in dermatopathology that help to diagnose and prognosticate melanoma. Clin Dermatol 2009;27:75–102.
11. Diwan AH, Dang SM, Prieto VG, et al. Lack of maturation with anti-leptin receptor antibody in melanoma. Mod Pathol 2009;22:103–6.

Dysplastic Nevi

Loren E. Clarke, MD[a,b,*]

KEYWORDS

• Dysplastic • Nevus • Atypical cytology • Clark's nevus
• Melanoma in situ

INTRODUCTION

The term dysplastic nevus was introduced soon after the description of the B-K mole syndrome by Wallace Clark and colleagues in 1978 to describe a common but clinically and histopathologically distinct type of melanocytic nevus.[1] The precise definition has been the source of great controversy, many synonyms have been proposed[2–4] (atypical nevus, Clark's nevus, nevus with architectural disorder, and melanocytic atypia), and although a National Institutes of Health Consensus Conference[5] once recommended against its use, the term dysplastic nevus is now widely used.[6] In a large survey of dermatologists, the dysplastic nevus was acknowledged as a distinct entity by 98% of responders.[7]

Patients with multiple dysplastic nevi have an increased risk for malignant melanoma,[8] and dysplastic nevi themselves have at least some potential for malignant transformation[7] in a manner somewhat analogous to that of adenomas of the colon.

Development of malignant melanoma is uncommon within dysplastic nevi, however. Since this transformation occurs in other types of nevi (eg, congenital nevi), their role as a marker of increased risk for melanoma in the patients who bear them seems to be their greater significance.[9,10]

GROSS OR CLINICAL FEATURES OF DYSPLASTIC NEVI

Dysplastic nevi are generally encountered in two clinical settings. In the first, referred to as dysplastic nevus syndrome or familial atypical multiple mole melanoma syndrome,[11–14] patients have numerous dysplastic nevi and a personal or family history of melanoma. Within the United States, familial dysplastic nevus syndrome probably affects approximately 32,000 individuals.[15] Far more common is the second setting, in which patients have a variable number of dysplastic nevi, perhaps only a few, and no strong family history of melanoma.

A version of this article was previously published in *Surgical Pathology Clinics* 2:3.

[a] Departments of Pathology, H179, The Penn State Hershey Medical Center, Hershey, PA 17033, USA

[b] Department of Dermatology, The Penn State Hershey Medical Center, Hershey, PA 17033, USA

* Department of Pathology, H179, The Penn State Hershey Medical Center, Hershey, PA 17033, USA.

E-mail address: lclarke@hmc.psu.edu

Clin Lab Med 31 (2011) 255–265
doi:10.1016/j.cll.2011.03.003
labmed.theclinics.com
0272-2712/11/$ – see front matter

Key Features
Dysplastic Nevi

Markers of increased risk for malignant melanoma, particularly in patients with multiple lesions

Occur sporadically and within a familial setting

Development of malignant melanoma within a dysplastic nevus is rare

Differential diagnosis includes superficial spreading melanoma and melanoma in situ

Histopathologic criteria for diagnosis and grading remain controversial and interobserver variability is significant

In a given individual, dysplastic nevi may be solitary or number in the hundreds. They are usually larger than other types of nevi, have irregular or ill-defined borders, and irregularly distributed pigment or pigment of multiple colors (**Figs. 1** and **2**).[1] They may be macules, papules, or plaques. The most common location is the trunk,[1] but they may occur at any anatomic site.

MICROSCOPIC FEATURES OF DYSPLASTIC NEVI

Dysplastic nevi exhibit a wide range of morphologic features and, despite numerous attempts at consensus, criteria that define dysplasia are not universally agreed upon, even among experts.[16] Generally accepted criteria, however, include (1) nevus cells arranged singly or in small nests along the tips and sides of rete ridges (**Fig. 3**); (2) fibroplasia of the papillary dermis (**Fig. 4**); (3) intraepidermal nevus cells extending horizontally more than 3 rete pegs beyond those in the dermis (shouldering) in lesions that are compound (**Fig. 5**); (4) a lymphohistiocytic inflammatory infiltrate; and (5) random cytologic atypia, including melanocytes with nuclear enlargement, prominent nucleoli, and expanded chromatin (**Fig. 6**).[7,16–18] Other types of nevi may also have a dysplastic component. For example, features of a dysplastic nevus are sometimes encountered within lesions that otherwise resemble a congenital-pattern nevus.[19]

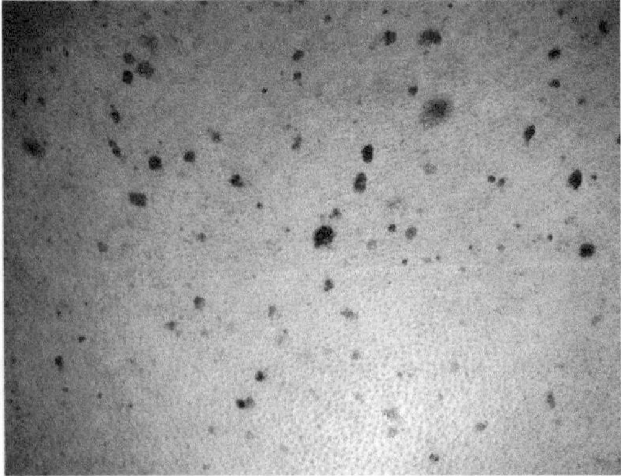

Fig. 1. Clinically, dysplastic nevi often exhibit irregular borders and irregularly distributed pigment. Many of the lesions are small. Some authors require that a nevus be greater than 5 mm in size to qualify as truly dysplastic. (*Courtesy of* Bryan Anderson, MD.)

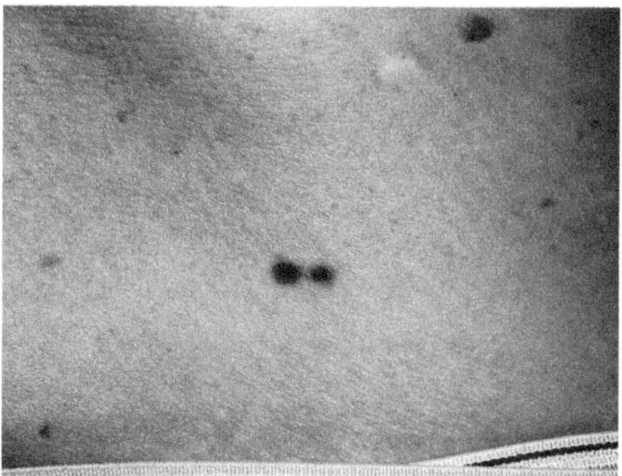

Fig. 2. The borders of dysplastic nevi are often described as ill defined or fuzzy. (*Courtesy of* Bryan Anderson, MD.)

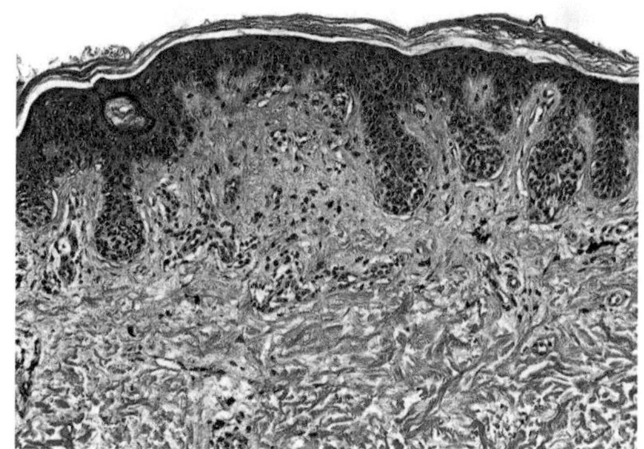

Fig. 3. Nevus cells are arranged singly and in small nests along the tips and sides of rete.

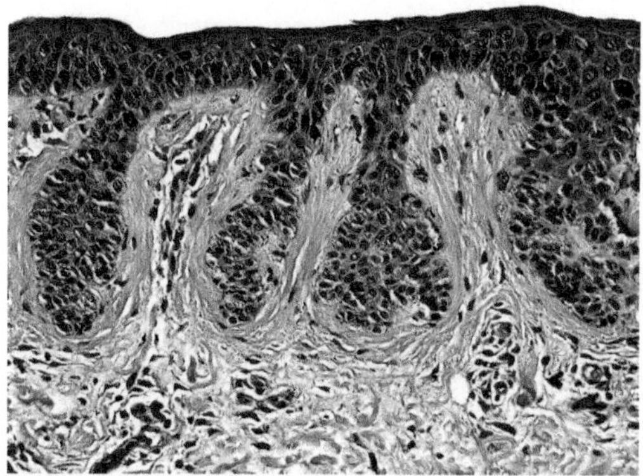

Fig. 4. There is dense lamellar fibrosis around the rete tips in this junctional dysplastic nevus.

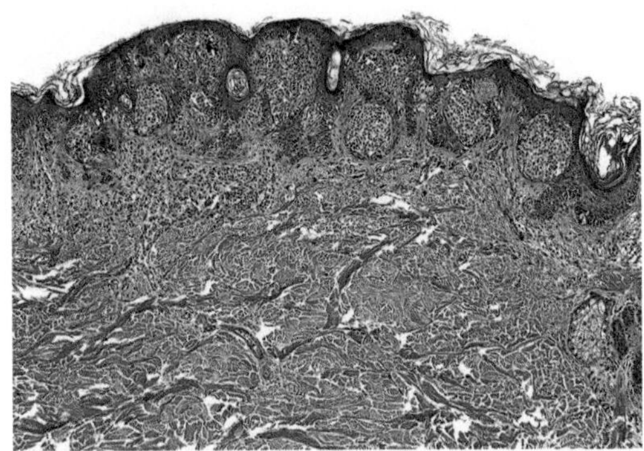

Fig. 5. This compound dysplastic nevus exhibits "shouldering": the lateral extension of the junctional component beyond the dermal component. Note also the lymphocytic infiltrate and pigment-containing macrophages.

More subjective is the grading of dysplasia within dysplastic nevi, for which many dermatopathologists employ a three-tiered system of mild, moderate, and severe.[20] Emphasis is often placed on cytologic features (**Figs. 7–9**). Weinstock and colleagues[21] outlined specific criteria that could be used to classify the atypia of intraepidermal melanocytes with reasonable reliability among multiple observers. For mild atypia, these included nuclear size similar to that of a basal keratinocyte, condensed chromatin, inconspicuous nucleoli, and scant cytoplasm. Moderate atypia was defined as nuclear size one to one and one-half times the basal keratinocyte nucleus, condensed or dispersed chromatin, inconspicuous nucleoli, and scant to abundant cytoplasm. Severe atypia was defined as nuclear size equal to or greater than twice that of a basal keratinocyte nucleus, marked nuclear pleomorphism (with some at least twice as large as others), dense hyperchromatism or dispersed chromatin with thickened nuclear membranes, prominent nucleoli, and scant to abundant cytoplasm. There remains little agreement about which criteria are most significant within grading schemes, and not surprisingly, interobserver reliability has been poor in some studies.[20,22–25] Nonetheless, degree of atypia

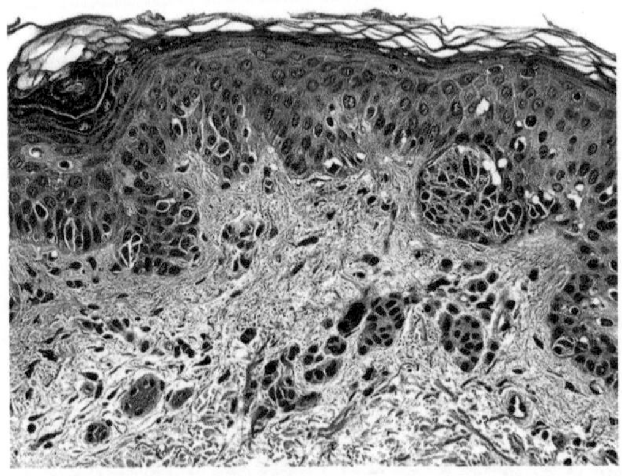

Fig. 6. This compound dysplastic nevus exhibits random cytologic atypia. The lesional melanocytes vary in size, shape, and chromatin distribution.

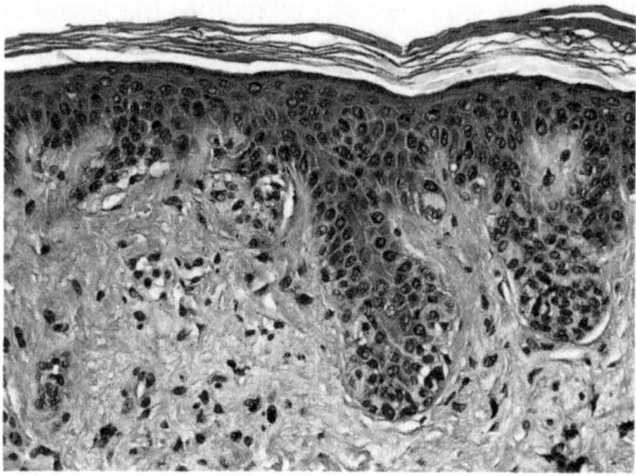

Fig. 7. Mild cytologic atypia. The nevus cells are generally equal in size to the adjacent basal layer keratinocytes and have uniformly distributed chromatin and inconspicuous nucleoli.

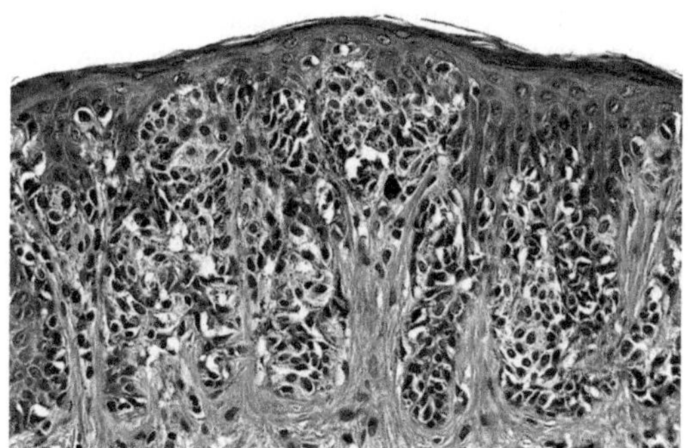

Fig. 8. Moderate cytologic atypia. Many of the lesional melanocytes are larger than adjacent keratinocytes and some contain conspicuous nucleoli.

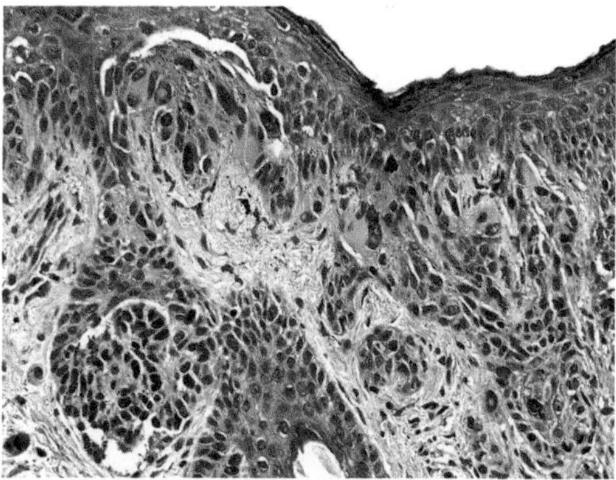

Fig. 9. Severe cytologic atypia. Several of the lesional cells within the center of the field contain nuclei that are more than twice the size of those within surrounding keratinocytes, and some exhibit marked nuclear hyperchromasia and irregular nuclear contours.

has been shown to correlate with risk of melanoma. Moderate or severe atypia in a dysplastic nevus has been associated with an increased risk of melanoma independent of confounding variables.[20,26] In comparison to mild dysplasia, nevi with moderate and severe dysplasia, as defined by Arumi-Uria and colleagues,[26] (1) exhibited less lateral circumscription, more asymmetry, rete ridge distortion, focal upward migration of nevus cells within the epidermis (primarily within the center of the lesion) (**Fig. 10**); (2) growth of nevus cells along interrete areas (ie, involvement of the suprapapillary plates) (**Fig. 11**) and (3) medium to large nuclear size, medium to large nucleoli, expanded or coarse chromatin pattern, and mitotic activity (**Fig. 12**).[26] It should be recognized that malignant melanomas share many of these features, albeit usually in a more exaggerated fashion.

Immunohistochemistry plays only a limited role in the evaluation of dysplastic nevi. Occasionally, a reliable and specific immunohistochemical marker of melanocytes may help highlight the distribution of lesional melanocytes, particularly the degree of upward pagetoid scatter of single melanocytes, when the cells are small and difficult to differentiate from epidermal keratinocytes. As with any immunohistochemical stain, selection is based on what stain performs well in a given laboratory. There are potential pitfalls with a variety of immunohistochemical stains used for recognizing melanocytes. This may be especially true with inflamed lesions, where immunohistochemical stains for Melan-A and HMB45 can falsely label keratinocytes, presumably owing to transfer of melanosomes to keratinocytes.[26] It may be prudent to consider the inclusion of immunohistochemical stains for S100 protein or microphthalmia transcription factor (MITF). With stains for S100 protein, care must be taken not to confuse Langerhans cells with pagetoid melanocytes. The presence of dendritic cytoplasmic processes can help, as pagetoid melanocytes typically lack that morphology. Positive stains for MITF highlight nuclei, potentially avoiding the pitfall with cytoplasmic stains.[27]

DIAGNOSIS OF DYSPLASTIC NEVI

While the diagnosis of dysplastic nevi may be made on histopathologic grounds alone, clinical information may be very helpful to the pathologist, and clinicians should be encouraged to provide at least a brief description of the lesions they biopsy. For example, a gross estimate of size may suggest whether a small biopsy is likely to be representative of the entire lesion, and pathologists may include a comment to

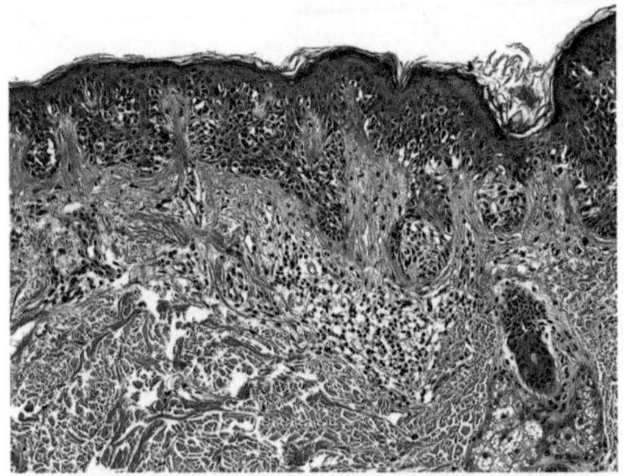

Fig. 10. Mild pagetoid scatter. There is upward spread of a few lesional cells to the mid stratum spinosum within this lesion.

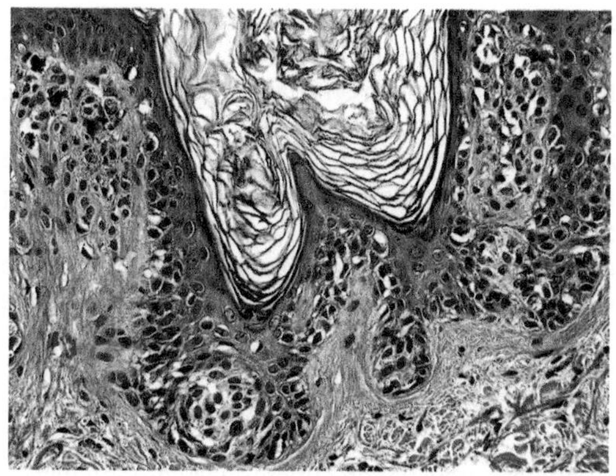

Fig. 11. Lentiginous growth. In addition to nest formation at the rete tips, there is spread of lesional melanocytes along the interrete areas (suprapapillary plates) in this dysplastic nevus.

this effect within a report. A clinical history that a lesion has recently changed or grown, or is of new onset, particularly in an older patient, may occasionally help a pathologist recognize that a borderline lesion is in fact melanoma rather than a dysplastic nevus.[28] Particularly helpful clinicians may describe specific portions of larger lesions that are suspicious, such as "nevus with peripherally-located black spot" or "central nodule." In this case, pathologists should be sure these specific areas are submitted for microscopic examination so the possibility of melanoma evolving within a nevus may be evaluated. Also important is a history of prior biopsy or excision of the lesion in question, since recurrent nevi often exhibit increased atypia and even mimic malignant melanoma. Pathologists should also be aware that not every clinically atypical nevus is a dysplastic nevus. Congenital nevi, nevus spilus, and other types of nevi may occasionally mimic a dysplastic nevus clinically.

There is usually little to be gained from gross examination of small, partial biopsies of dysplastic nevi, but inspection of larger excision specimens (or high-quality photographs of them) before submission for microscopy may reveal diagnostically useful information, including adequacy of sampling (if the lesion is not entirely submitted) and distance of the lesion from margins.

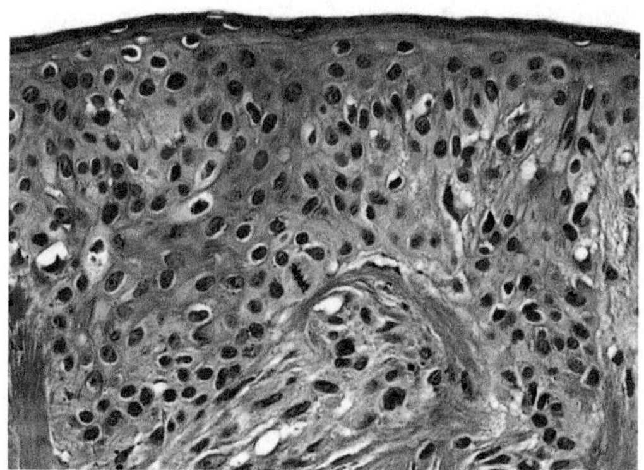

Fig. 12. A mitotic figure is present within a junctional melanocyte.

In general, pathology reports describing dysplastic nevi may indicate the grade of dysplasia and whether the lesion is junctional or compound. Pathologists may comment on margin involvement, even on shave or punch biopsies of nevi, since clinicians sometimes perform these procedures intending to wholly remove the lesion.[29] However, this should be done with the understanding by pathologist and clinician (and ultimately the patient) that margin interpretation in these biopsies may not be as reliable as for formal excisions.

As mentioned, some dysplastic nevi exhibit substantial histopathologic overlap with early superficial spreading melanoma or melanoma in situ and, in rare instances, reliable distinction cannot be made. In such cases, pathologists may provide a descriptive diagnosis such as "atypical compound melanocytic proliferation" with a comment stating that malignancy cannot be excluded and that complete excision of the lesion is recommended.

Management of dysplastic nevi varies substantially among clinicians.[7] Most recognize that a diagnosis of dysplastic nevus often signifies at least some increased risk of melanoma for the patient and, possibly, for the patient's relatives, and will perform a careful and thorough skin examination and evaluation of family history if this has not already been done. Some will completely re-excise a dysplastic nevus of any grade, while others will do so only for nevi designated moderately or severely dysplastic. Many will weigh the various clinical and practical factors that come into play and make decisions on a case-by-case basis, usually with input from the patient.

PROGNOSIS OF DYSPLASTIC NEVI

The incidence of melanoma arising from or in association with a dysplastic nevus is difficult to define but has been estimated at 1:3000 per year.[30] The majority of dysplastic nevi remain stable over time, and some even regress.[28] In light of this low frequency of malignant progression, the primary significance of a dysplastic nevus is its ability to identify those at increased risk for melanoma at other sites. Patients with numerous dysplastic nevi are at a greater risk for melanoma,[31] and dysplastic nevi are one of the strongest risk factors for melanoma.[8,32]

DIFFERENTIAL DIAGNOSIS OF DYSPLASTIC NEVI

Malignant Melanoma

Malignant melanoma is obviously the most important differential diagnostic consideration. In general, dysplastic nevi exhibit symmetry, lateral borders that are well-circumscribed relative to those of melanoma, uniformity in the size and shape of melanocytic nests, equidistant spacing of nests, and an absence of upward spread of melanocytes (pagetoid spread) into the spinous and granular layers of the epidermis. In compound variants, the dermal melanocytes of a nevus should exhibit evidence of senescence or maturation, including gradually diminishing nuclear size and cytoplasmic volume with progressive descent into the dermis, and dispersion (ie, the distribution of nevus cells as solitary units rather than cell clusters or aggregates). Cytologic atypia is generally more pronounced within melanoma, and the observation of two distinctly different populations of melanocytes within a lesion may indicate melanoma arising within a pre-existing nevus.

Congenital Nevus

Portions of congenital nevi may exhibit histopathologic features that overlap with those of a dysplastic nevus. In general, congenital nevi may be recognized by their tendency to exhibit nevus cells in close association with adnexal structures and to

Differential Diagnosis
Dysplastic Nevi

- Malignant melanoma
  - Dysplastic nevi
    - Symmetry, lateral borders well-circumscribed relative to melanoma
    - Uniformity in the size and shape of melanocytic nests and equidistant spacing
    - Absence of upward spread of melanocytes into epidermis
  - Compound variants of dysplastic nevi
    - Dermal melanocytes exhibit evidence of senescence or maturation, dispersion, distribution of nevus cells as solitary units rather than cell clusters or aggregates
  - Within pre-existing nevus
    - Two distinctly different populations of melanocytes within a lesion may indicate melanoma arising
- Congenital nevus
  - Tendency to exhibit nevus cells closely associated with adnexal structures
  - Extend into the reticular dermis with nevus cells splaying among individual dermal collagen bundles
- Recurrent nevus
  - Junctional component usually exhibits extensive lentiginous growth of single melanocytes
  - Sharp localization of melanocytic proliferation above a scar is evidence supporting a recurrent nevus

extend into the reticular dermis with nevus cells splaying among individual dermal collagen bundles. Nonetheless, dysplastic nevi that also exhibit congenital features are common. These may be designated combined nevi, with features of dysplastic and congenital nevi.

Recurrent Nevus

Recurrent nevi of many types may mimic a dysplastic nevus or a melanoma since the junctional component usually exhibits extensive lentiginous growth of single

Pitfalls
Dysplastic Nevi

! Dysplastic nevi are uncommon on the face. A diagnosis of lentigo maligna (melanoma in situ) or other form of melanoma must be carefully excluded—especially when evidence of sun damage is present—before diagnosing a facial dysplastic nevus. Dysplastic nevi in severely sun-damaged skin in other locations should also be viewed with heightened suspicion for melanoma

! Nevi in acral skin, genital skin, and breast skin (so-called special sites) may exhibit increased architectural atypia that must not be over-interpreted as severe dysplasia or melanoma. In acral sites, this may include upward spread of single melanocytes into the spinous and even granular layers of the epidermis

! Recurrent nevi may mimic a dysplastic nevus or melanoma since the junctional component often exhibits increased architectural disorder, including extensive lentiginous growth of single melanocytes. Sharp localization of the melanocytic proliferation to the area above a scar is evidence in support of a recurrent nevus

melanocytes. Sharp localization of the melanocytic proliferation to the area above a scar is evidence in support of a recurrent nevus.

REFERENCES

1. Clark WH Jr, Reimer RR, Greene M, et al. Origin of familial malignant melanomas from heritable melanocytic lesions. 'The B-K mole syndrome'. Arch Dermatol 1978;114(5):732–8.
2. Ackerman AB. What naevus is dysplastic, a syndrome and the commonest precursor of malignant melanoma? A riddle and an answer. Histopathology 1988;13(3):241–56.
3. Glusac EJ. What to call the LEJC-BFV nevus? J Cutan Pathol 2004;31(8):521–2.
4. Ackerman AB, Magana-Garcia M. Naming acquired melanocytic nevi. Unna's, Miescher's, Spitz's Clark's. Am J Dermatopathol 1990;12(2):193–209.
5. NIH Consensus Conference. Diagnosis and treatment of early melanoma. JAMA 1992;268(10):1314–9.
6. Shapiro M, Chren MM, Levy RM, et al. Variability in nomenclature used for nevi with architectural disorder and cytologic atypia (microscopically dysplastic nevi) by dermatologists and dermatopathologists. J Cutan Pathol 2004;31(8):523–30.
7. Tripp JM, Kopf AW, Marghoob AA, et al. Management of dysplastic nevi: a survey of fellows of the American Academy of Dermatology. J Am Acad Dermatol 2002; 46(5):674–82.
8. Gandini S, Sera F, Cattaruzza MS, et al. Meta-analysis of risk factors for cutaneous melanoma: I. Common and atypical naevi. Eur J Cancer 2005;41(1):28–44.
9. Carey WP Jr, Thompson CJ, Synnestvedt M, et al. Dysplastic nevi as a melanoma risk factor in patients with familial melanoma. Cancer 1994;74(12):3118–25.
10. Halpern AC, Guerry DT, Elder DE, et al. Dysplastic nevi as risk markers of sporadic (nonfamilial) melanoma. A case-control study. Arch Dermatol 1991; 127(7):995–9.
11. Lynch HT, Frichot BC 3rd, Lynch JF. Familial atypical multiple mole-melanoma syndrome. J Med Genet 1978;15(5):352–6.
12. Lynch HT, Fusaro RM, Lynch JF. A medical and genetic critique of the familial atypical multiple mole melanoma syndrome and the dysplastic nevus syndrome. Am J Dermatopathol 1985;7(Suppl):S107–16.
13. Lynch HT, Fusaro RM, Pester J, et al. Familial atypical multiple mole melanoma (FAMMM) syndrome: genetic heterogeneity and malignant melanoma. Br J Cancer 1980;42(1):58–70.
14. Lynch HT, Fusaro RM, Treger CL, et al. The cutaneous evolution of nevi in a patient with familial, atypical, multiple-mole melanoma syndrome. Pediatr Dermatol 1985; 2(4):289–93.
15. Kraemer KH, Greene MH, Tarone R, et al. Dysplastic naevi and cutaneous melanoma risk. Lancet 1983;2(8358):1076–7.
16. Roth ME, Grant-Kels JM, Ackerman AB, et al. The histopathology of dysplastic nevi. Continued controversy. Am J Dermatopathol 1991;13(1):38–51.
17. Kelly JW, Crutcher WA, Sagebiel RW. Clinical diagnosis of dysplastic melanocytic nevi. A clinicopathologic correlation. J Am Acad Dermatol 1986;14(6):1044–52.
18. Rhodes AR, Mihm MC Jr, Weinstock MA. Dysplastic melanocytic nevi: a reproducible histologic definition emphasizing cellular morphology. Mod Pathol 1989;2(4): 306–19.
19. Toussaint S, Kamino H. Dysplastic changes in different types of melanocytic nevi. A unifying concept. J Cutan Pathol 1999;26(2):84–90.

20. Shors AR, Kim S, White E, et al. Dysplastic naevi with moderate to severe histological dysplasia: a risk factor for melanoma. Br J Dermatol 2006;155(5):988–93.
21. Weinstock MA, Barnhill RL, Rhodes AR, et al. Reliability of the histopathologic diagnosis of melanocytic dysplasia. The Dysplastic Nevus Panel. Arch Dermatol 1997;133(8):953–8.
22. Piepkorn MW, Barnhill RL, Cannon-Albright LA, et al. A multiobserver, population-based analysis of histologic dysplasia in melanocytic nevi. J Am Acad Dermatol 1994;30(5 Pt 1):707–14.
23. Duncan LM, Berwick M, Bruijn JA, et al. Histopathologic recognition and grading of dysplastic melanocytic nevi: an interobserver agreement study. J Invest Dermatol 1993;100(3):318S–21S.
24. Lodha S, Saggar S, Celebi JT, et al. Discordance in the histopathologic diagnosis of difficult melanocytic neoplasms in the clinical setting. J Cutan Pathol 2008; 35(4):349–52.
25. Farmer ER, Gonin R, Hanna MP. Discordance in the histopathologic diagnosis of melanoma and melanocytic nevi between expert pathologists. Hum Pathol 1996; 27(6):528–31.
26. Arumi-Uria M, McNutt NS, Finnerty B. Grading of atypia in nevi: correlation with melanoma risk. Mod Pathol 2003;16(8):764–71.
27. Maize JC Jr, Resneck JS Jr, Shapiro PE, et al. Ducking stray "magic bullets": a Melan-A alert. Am J Dermatopathol 2003;25(2):162–5.
28. Tucker MA, Fraser MC, Goldstein AM, et al. A natural history of melanomas and dysplastic nevi: an atlas of lesions in melanoma-prone families. Cancer 2002; 94(12):3192–209.
29. Sellheyer K, Bergfeld WF, Stewart E, et al. Evaluation of surgical margins in melanocytic lesions: a survey among 152 dermatopathologists. J Cutan Pathol 2005; 32(4):293–9.
30. Cockerell CJG-KJ, Canther JC, LeBoit P. Pathology and genetics of skin tumours. Lyon: IARC Press; 2006.
31. Holly EA, Kelly JW, Shpall SN, et al. Number of melanocytic nevi as a major risk factor for malignant melanoma. J Am Acad Dermatol 1987;17(3):459–68.
32. Tucker MA, Halpern A, Holly EA, et al. Clinically recognized dysplastic nevi. A central risk factor for cutaneous melanoma. JAMA 1997;277(18):1439–44.

Congenital Melanocytic Nevi

Maya Zayour, MD[a], Rossitza Lazova, MD[b,*]

KEYWORDS

• Congenital • Nevus • Melanoma • Nevoid • Melanocytic

OVERVIEW: CONGENITAL MELANOCYTIC NEVI

Congenital melanocytic nevi (CMN) are melanocytic nevi that have their onset at birth or shortly thereafter and show distinct histopathologic features. CMN differ from common acquired nevi by their overall size, depth of involvement by nevus cells, and adnexal and vascular involvement. Not uncommonly, however, melanocytic nevi in adults show similar histologic characteristics without a supporting clinical history of a congenital onset and are sometimes designated as melanocytic nevi with congenital features.

CMN may be classified according to their size as small (diameter <1.5 cm), medium (diameter 1.5 to 20 cm), or large/giant (diameter >20 cm). CMN are relatively common with an incidence among newborns ranging between 0.2% and 6%.[1,2] Giant congenital nevi are rare, with an estimated incidence of 0.0005%.[3] They can also be classified according to the location of the melanocytic proliferation: junctional, compound, or intradermal.

Accurate estimates of melanoma risk associated with CMN are difficult to obtain.[3] The potential risk is related to the size of the CMN—that is, the larger the nevus, the greater the risk. In general, small and medium CMN are not associated with significant risk for developing melanoma.[4,5] A lifetime risk of approximately 6.3% has been estimated from the Danish Birth Registry.[6] DeDavid and colleagues[7] analyzed the world literature and found that out of 289 patients with large CMN, 12% developed primary cutaneous melanoma within their nevi.

GROSS FEATURES

Small CMN may be indistinguishable from common acquired nevi and documentation at birth may be the only means of confirming a congenital origin. In general, small and

A version of this article was previously published in *Surgical Pathology Clinics* 2:3.
[a] Yale Dermatopathology Laboratory, Department of Dermatology, Yale University School of Medicine, 15 York Street, PO Box 208059, New Haven, CT 06520, USA
[b] Department of Dermatology and Pathology, Yale University School of Medicine, 15 York Street, PO Box 208059, New Haven, CT 06520, USA
* Corresponding author.
E-mail address: rossitza.lazova@yale.edu

Clin Lab Med 31 (2011) 267–280
doi:10.1016/j.cll.2011.03.004 **labmed.theclinics.com**
0272-2712/11/$ – see front matter

Key Features
Pathologic key features: congenital melanocytic nevi

1. Symmetric proliferation of melanocytes with a V-shaped or plate-like dermal component
2. Well circumscribed junctional component with regularly spaced and relatively monomorphous melanocytic nests
3. Extension of nevus cells into deep reticular dermis and subcutis
4. Maturation of melanocytes with their descent
5. Tracking of melanocytes around and within appendages, vessels, or nerves
6. Splaying of collagen bundles by nevus cells arranged in single rows or cords

medium-sized CMN are well delineated, round, elongate, or oval. CMN may be flat (macular); elevated (papular); verrucous; or, rarely, cerebriform.[8] They vary in color from tan to dark brown to black and are usually evenly pigmented. Coarse dark hairs with an increased density are often present.

Gross examination of excisional biopsies of congenital nevi should be performed carefully. It is important to ensure, particularly in medium and large CMN, that all darker, elevated, unusual appearing, and suspicious areas are sampled for microscopic examination. Gross features to cause concern include:

1. An outgrowth peripheral to the outline of the main nevus or vertical as a palpable nodule
2. An ill-defined border indistinctly blending with the surrounding nonlesional skin
3. A focus of hypo- or hyperpigmentation diverging from the general uniform color of the nevus.

Because staged excision is a common modality for management of large congenital nevi, pathologists may get multiple sequential specimens from the same lesion on one or several occasions; all specimens from a patient should be amply sampled with attention to the features listed previously.

MICROSCOPIC FEATURES OF CONGENITAL MELANOCYTIC NEVI

CMN may be junctional, compound, or exclusively intradermal. The histologic characteristics are related primarily to the size of the nevus. There is a striking correlation between nevus size and nevus depth, which seems to be established very early in life.[9] Small CMN may be entirely junctional and indistinguishable from acquired nevi.[9] Many small CMN demonstrate a superficial congenital pattern, which refers to nevus cells extending to no greater depth than the upper half of the reticular dermis, and some small CMN may not show the classic histologic features of CMN as originally outlined by Mark and colleagues.[10] These features include

1. Extension of nevus cells into the deep reticular dermis and sometimes into the superficial subcutaneous fat
2. Tracking of melanocytes around or within appendageal, vascular, and neural structures
3. Involvement of reticular dermis by nevus cells arranged as single cells, rows (files), cords (double rows), and sheets of cells splaying in between dermal collagen bundles.

At scanning magnification, CMN are usually symmetric with a V- (wedge-)shaped or plate-like dermal component (**Fig. 1**). If a junctional component is present, it is well circumscribed (ie, the nevus starts with a nest of melanocytes on one side and ends with a nest on the other side). Nests of melanocytes positioned at sides and bases of rete ridges are evenly distributed, relatively uniform in size and shape, and predominate over single melanocytes (**Fig. 2**). The melanocytes are typically small to medium and are monomorphous. In compound CMN, in addition to a junctional component, there are nevus cells in the dermis, which tend to be aggregated in nests. Melanocytes are larger in the most superficial portion of the dermis. They are uniform, with scant cytoplasm, and show maturation from the superficial to the deep aspect of the lesion with nests of melanocytes and individual melanocytes gradually diminishing in size with their descent into the dermis. With increasing depth, the nevus cells often demonstrate less crowding and greater splaying of the collagen (see **Fig. 2**). Occasional mitotic figures may be noted in CMN, usually in the superficial portion of the lesion.[11]

With increasing size, there is a greater tendency for deep dermal, appendageal, and neurovascular involvement.[9] In large CMN, there is a diffuse proliferation of nevus cells throughout the reticular dermis with frequent extension into the subcutis.[9,10] Nevus cells often extend along fibrous septae of the subcutaneous fat and, in some instances, may infiltrate the fat lobules. Aggregates of nevus cells tend to cuff or be present within follicular epithelium, sebaceous glands, eccrine ducts and glands, the perineurium of nerve twigs, walls of vessels, and pilar erector muscles (**Figs. 3** and **4**).[9,10,12] A subset of large CMN is also characterized by spindle cell or neural differentiation with nevus cells with wavy configuration resembling the histologic pattern of a neurofibroma.[13]

DIFFERENTIAL DIAGNOSIS FOR CONGENITAL MELANOCYTIC NEVI

Nevoid Melanoma

Nevoid melanoma (see article by [Smith and colleagues] elsewhere in this issue) often resembles a compound or predominantly intradermal melanocytic nevus with features of CMN. Architectural features that should raise suspicion of a nevoid melanoma are asymmetry, prominent cellular density, and scatter of melanocytes throughout the epidermis. It is essential, however, to be aware that some upward migration of

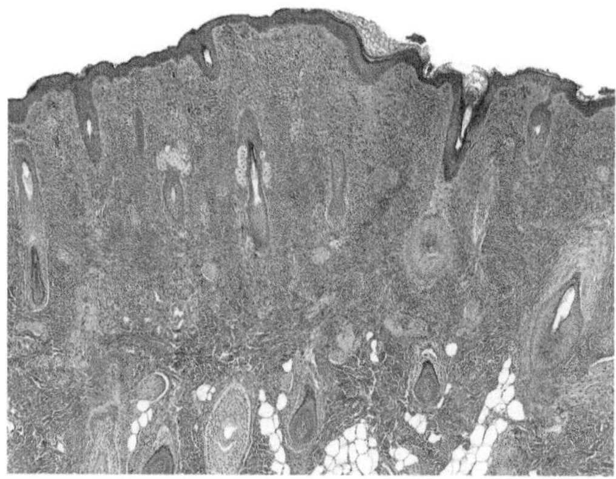

Fig. 1. Low-power magnification of a congenital nevus with a symmetric outline and maturation of melanocytes with their descent.

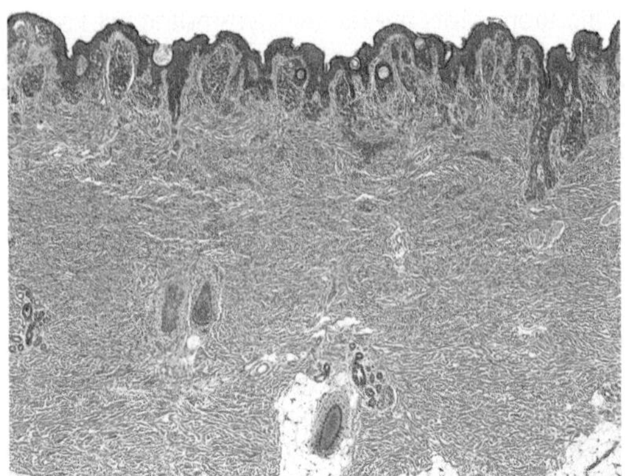

Fig. 2. Compound congenital melanocytic nevus showing prominent splaying of nevus cells in between collagen bundles in the dermis.

melanocytes is a common finding in CMN, particularly in neonates and young children. In CMN, however, the pagetoid melanocytes show at most only mild cytologic atypia, do not extend beyond the dermal component, and involve the lower half of the epidermis without reaching the granular layer.[2] At higher magnification, the melanocytes of a nevoid melanoma show cytologic atypia with subtle pleomorphism, nuclear hyperchromasia, prominent nucleoli, coarse and "dusty" pigmentation of the cytoplasm (particularly of melanocytes in the deep portion of the lesion), and absence of maturation with dermal descent. The presence of mitotic figures in the deep aspects of the lesion or atypical mitotic figures favors nevoid melanoma. Occasionally, the use of ancillary studies, such as immunohistochemistry, may also provide additional useful information. In general the proliferative index Ki-67 and the proteins p53, p21, Rb, and Cyclin D show higher expression in nevoid melanoma whereas p16 shows lower immunolabeling in melanoma in comparsion of congenital nevi.[14] In some cases, comparative genomic hybridization may also prove helpful.[15,16]

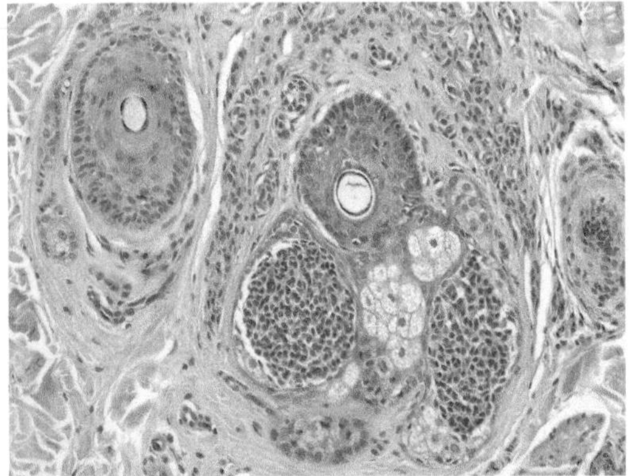

Fig. 3. Nevus cells are present within sebaceous lobules and surround the hair follicle. They are small and monomorphous.

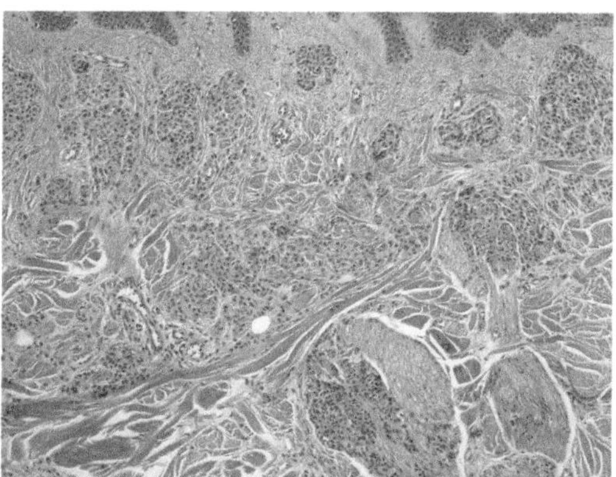

Fig. 4. Melanocytes are seen within arrector pilar muscles.

Malignant Melanoma Developing in Congenital Nevi

Melanomas may originate in small and medium-sized CMN with onset usually after puberty and peaking during ages 20 to 30 and 50 to 60 years. They often develop at the periphery of the pre-existing nevus. Virtually all melanomas have an intraepidermal origin and are usually of the conventional type.[17,18] Such melanomas are uncommonly observed in large/giant CMN, however; the majority of melanomas that develop in this setting are dermal. They present as relatively cohesive nodules that are distinctly different form the surrounding banal nevus (**Fig. 5**). These nodules tend to demonstrate marked cellularity and often have prominent nuclear pleomorphism, necrotic cells, and mitotic figures, including atypical forms.[18,19] The malignant melanocytes may be epithelioid, spindled, or small round cells with high nuclear-to-cytoplasmic ratio (**Fig. 6**).[18,19] The evaluation of such tumors may be difficult, and it may not always be possible to arrive at a definitive diagnosis of malignancy or benignancy. Because melanoma in newborns and infants younger than age 1 year is rare,

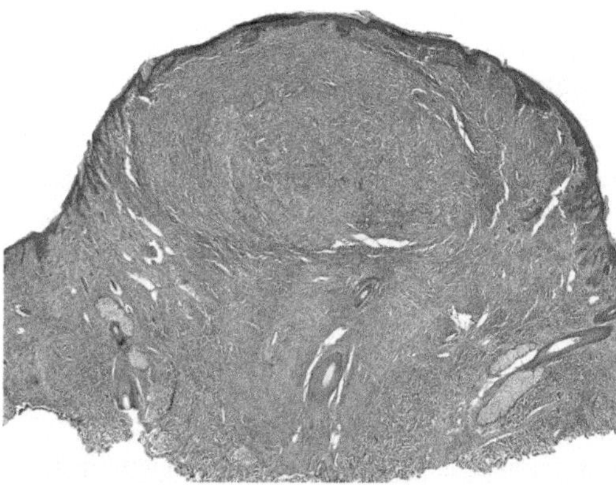

Fig. 5. In the background of a compound congenital melanocytic nevus with a wedge-shaped configuration is a centrally located nodule of melanoma, which blends with the surrounding nevus and makes the lesion asymmetric.

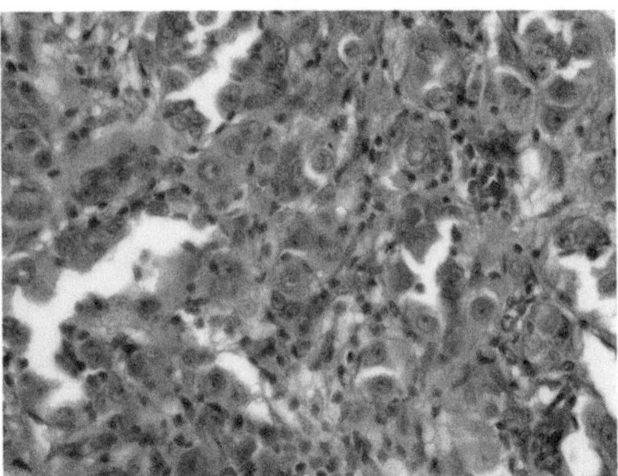

Fig. 6. Large pleomorphic melanocytes with irregular vesicular nuclei, prominent purple nucleoli, and abundant pale cytoplasm. Numerous lymphocytes are admixed with the neoplastic melanocytes.

a diagnosis of melanoma in young children should be rendered with extreme caution.[19] Furthermore, the majority of nodular melanocytic proliferations developing in CMN, particularly in neonates, represent proliferative nodules that behave in a benign fashion.

Melanocytic Nevi with Dysplastic and Congenital Features

Pathologists should be aware that dysplastic nevi might show a congenital pattern. One study suggests an incidence of 8.3% of compound dysplastic nevi having congenital features.[20] The classic histologic features of dysplastic nevi (see article by [Smith and colleagues] elsewhere in this issue) are present at the dermal epidermal junction and in the papillary dermis and include

1. Lentiginous melanocytic hyperplasia
2. Extension of the junctional component beyond the dermal component ("shoulders")
3. Junctional nests with variable sizes and shapes
4. Bridging between rete ridges
5. Confluence of nests
6. Lamellar and concentric fibroplasia in the papillary dermis
7. Variable cytologic atypia.

None of the above features is by itself diagnostic of dysplasia in a nevus with congenital features. Lentiginous melanocytic hyperplasia is often seen in CMN and more commonly in infants (**Fig. 7**).[10,12] Categorizing a given nevus as congenital with dysplastic features or as dyplastic nevus with features of a congenital nevus can be arbitrary.

DIAGNOSIS

Making a diagnosis of a congenital melanocytic nevus is usually not difficult when all histologic features are present, namely, symmetry, good circumscription, uniform nests in the epidermis equidistant from each other, nests of melanocytes and individual melanocytes that mature with their descent into the dermis, wrapping of nevus

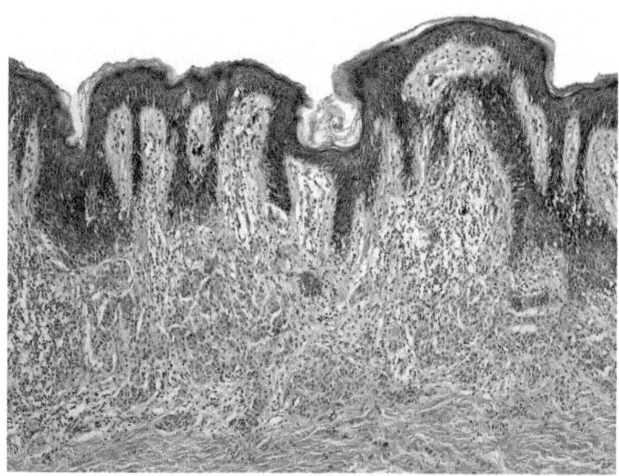

Fig. 7. In this congenital melanocytic nevus, there is prominent lentiginous melanocytic hyperplasia with single melanocytes and small nests of melanocytes present at the dermal epidermal junction. The nests are seen at bases and sides of rete ridges and, focally, there is bridging between adjacent rete ridges. Monomorphous melanocytes that mature with their descent are present in the dermis.

cells around vessels and adnexal structures, and splaying of melanocytes in between collagen bundles. Since the histopathologic findings are not always classic, pitfalls in the diagnosis of congenital melanocytic nevi include: lentiginous melanocytic proliferation, pagetoid scatter of melanocytes, proliferative nodules, and persistent/recurrent nevus.

Lentiginous melanocytic proliferation

One of the most common findings in CMN is the presence of lentiginous melanocytic proliferation, which may or may not be associated with variation in the size and shape of junctional melanocytic nests and the presence of some degree of cytologic atypia (see **Fig. 7**).[9] The junctional component of CMN, particularly in congenital nevi in individuals less than 10 years of age and especially in the first year of life and in certain

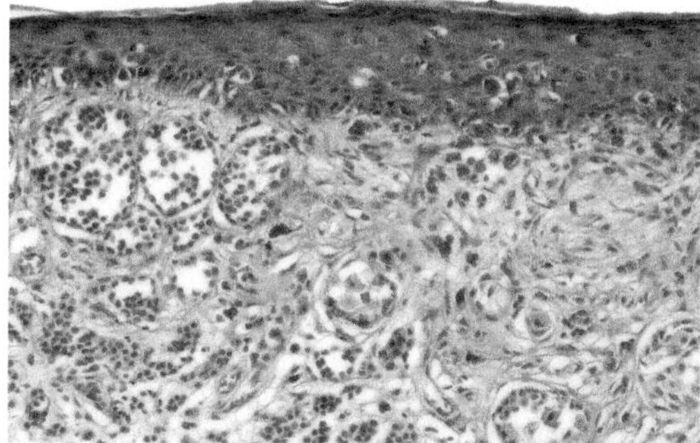

Fig. 8. In this congenital melanocytic nevus from a very young child, there is prominent pagetoid spread of melanocytes mainly in the lower portion of the epidermis. Nests of relatively monomorphous melanocytes are seen in the dermis.

locations, such as the scalp, may show large nests of melanocytes that vary in size and shape and that are not uniformly distributed. Single cells may predominate over nests in some high power fields and the melanocytes may be large, showing slight pleomorphism (**Fig. 8**). These findings may be misconstrued for those of malignant melanoma in situ. However, melanoma is rare in children, particularly in the setting of a preexisting nevus, which otherwise shows characteristic histopathologic features of CMN.

Pagetoid scatter of melanocytes

A common finding, particularly in children under the age of 10 and especially during the first year of life, is the presence of melanocytes above the dermal epidermal junction. The scatter of melanocytes, however, is usually confined to the lower half of the epidermis, the lesion appears symmetric, the proliferation of melanocytes is relatively orderly, and cytologic atypia is absent (see **Fig. 8**).[9,21,22]

Proliferative nodules in congenital nevi

Large/giant CMN or, rarely, melanocytic nevi, congenital or acquired, of any size, may give rise to intradermal nodular melanocytic proliferations. The majority of these proliferative nodules, particularly in the neonatal period, are biologically benign despite atypical histologic features. Such proliferations may occur in the superficial or deep reticular dermis, have a nodular configuration, and are comprised of epithelioid, spindled, or small melanocytes (**Fig. 9**). Often, the large epithelioid melanocytes have granular pigmented cytoplasm and uniform nuclei with evenly dispersed chromatin (**Fig. 10**).

Histologic features that differentiate a proliferative nodule from melanoma include[23]

1. Gradual blending of the melanocytes in the nodule with the surrounding nevus cells, reminiscent of maturation
2. Absence of destructive expansile growth

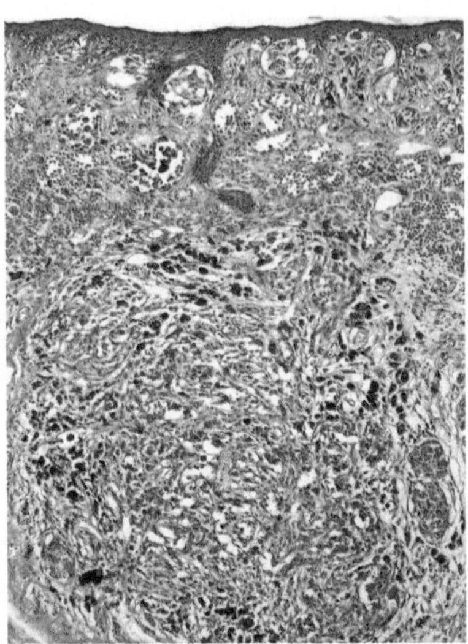

Fig. 9. Small and monomorphous melanocytes with scant cytoplasm are seen in the most superficial portion of the reticular dermis. Beneath that area is a well-defined nodule of much larger nested melanocytes with abundant and heavily pigmented cytoplasm.

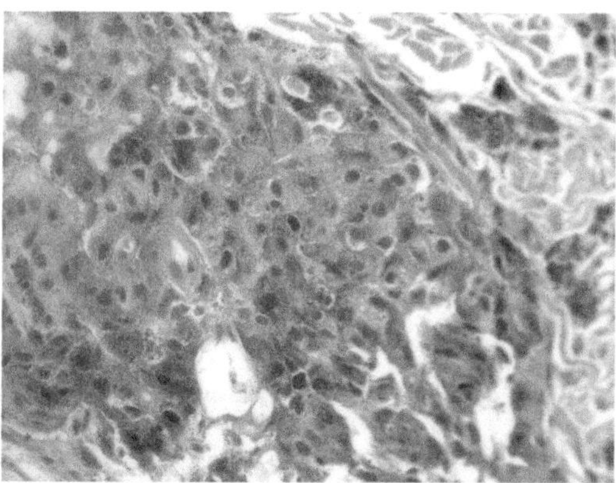

Fig. 10. Large melanocytes with abundant dusty pigmented cytoplasm and melanophages in the vicinity.

3. Absence of necrosis within the nodule
4. Absence of pagetoid spread in the overlying epidermis
5. Absence of severe and uniform cytologic atypia
6. Rare mitotic figures and absence of atypical mitoses.

Comparative genomic hybridization may be helpful in differentiating a proliferative nodule from melanoma arising in a congenital melanocytic nevus.[16,24]

Recurrent/persistent nevus

Sometimes, a variably irregular pigmentation arises confined to the site of a previously removed nevus or a biopsy site, worrisome clinically for atypia or melanoma. Histologic examination reveals often an irregular intraepidermal melanocytic proliferation confined to the area above a dermal scar with effacement of the rete ridges (**Figs. 11** and **12**). There is usually no or mild cytologic atypia and melanocytes may be

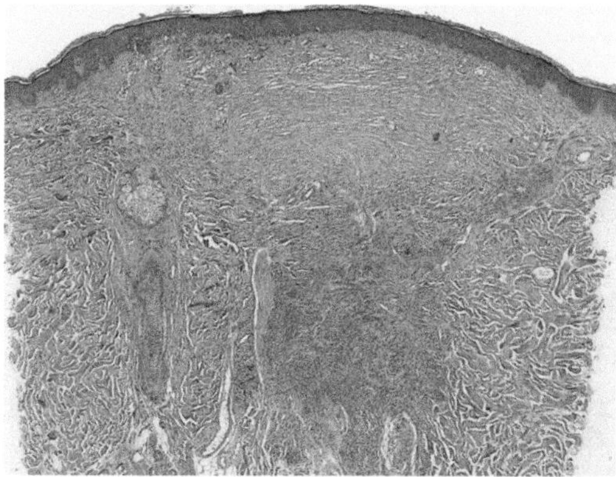

Fig. 11. This small congenital melanocytic nevus extending to the midreticular dermis has been previously sampled. A scar with collagen bundles and fibroblasts oriented parallel to the skin surface is seen immediately beneath the epidermis and above small banal nevus cells in the dermis.

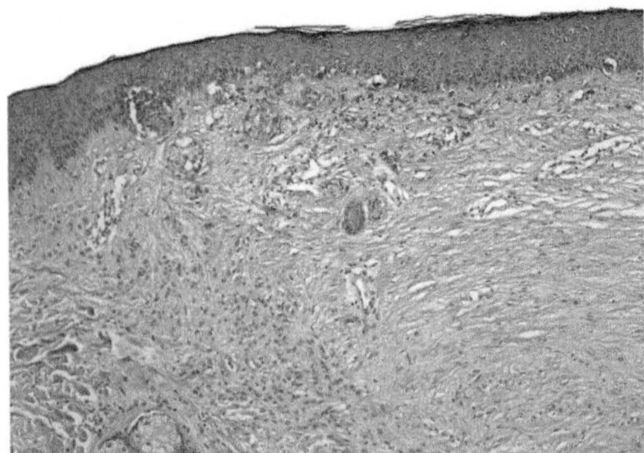

Fig. 12. A higher magnification of this recurrent nevus reveals a small number of monomorphous melanocytes in the dermis to the left of the scar. There are a few nests of melanocytes at the dermal epidermal junction and in the papillary dermis. In addition, single melanocytes in an irregular pattern are seen at the junction with rare melanocytes above it. These melanocytes have prominent pigment in their cytoplasm.

seen above the dermal epidermal junction, in the lower half of the epidermis (see **Fig. 12**). Remnants of the nevus may be present beneath the scar or peripherally, if the nevus was not completely removed (ie, persistent nevus) (**Figs. 13** and **14**). Knowing the clinical history of a prior intervention at this site, the confinement of the irregular intraepidermal proliferation to the area overlying the scar in the dermis, and often the presence of a residual banal nevus with congenital features, allows a distinction from melanoma in situ or melanoma, rendering a correct diagnosis of recurrent/ persistent nevus.[25–29]

PROGNOSIS

The risk of developing melanoma in congenital nevi is proportional to the size of the nevus. The exact incidence is unknown but ranges between 5% and 10% over

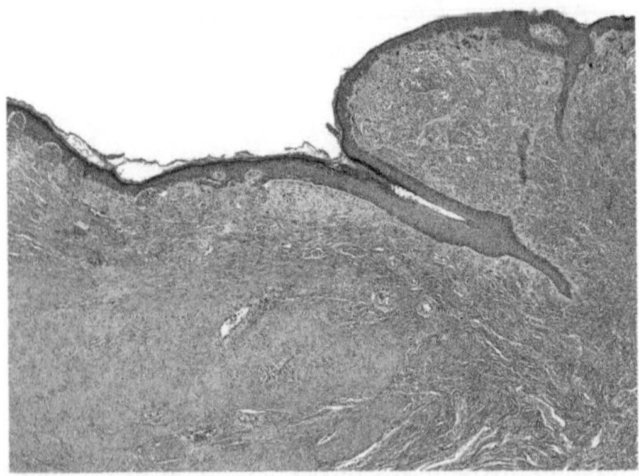

Fig. 13. A predominantly intradermal congenital melanocytic nevus that has been previously sampled, evidenced by the prominent scar in the dermis in the center and the left portion of the photomicrograph.

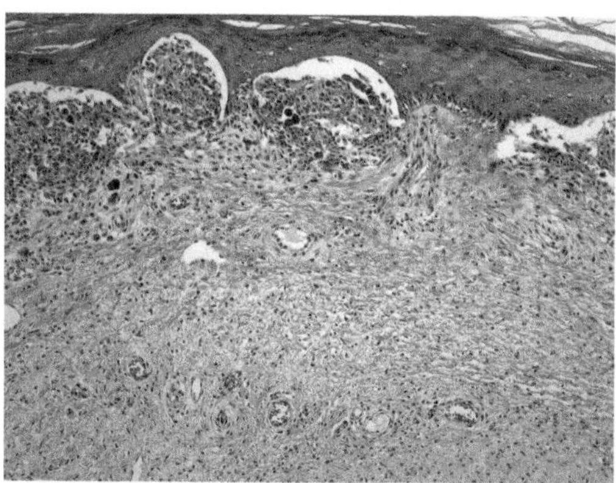

Fig. 14. Irregular, focally confluent nests of melanocytes displaying variation in their size and shape. Focal clefting is present between the nests and the adjacent epidermis. In addition, single melanocytes are also noted at the dermal epidermal junction with occasional melanocytes above it.

a lifetime for large nevi (more than 20 cm).[30] The risk of melanoma developing in association with small CMN (<1.5 cm) is not well established with one study suggesting a cumulative risk of between 2.6% and 4.9% for people who live to age 60.[31] Extremely rarely melanoma may be present at birth, or it may arise in infancy or later on, with most cases occurring within the first decade of life.[32,33] Melanomas arising in congenital nevi may show alarming cellularity and atypical features but they may not necessarily behave aggressively, especially in cases developing in the first few months of life.[18,34] Patients who develop melanoma should be closely followed as this deadly malignancy is notorious for an unpredictable behavior, including very late metastases.[35]

Changes within congenital nevi may be worrisome clinically and prompt clinicians to sample the nevus. Among the causes for a changing mole clinically are a rupture of a hair follicle or a cyst,[36,37] trauma,[38] infection,[39,40] development of a dermatofibroma,[41] or seborrheic keratosis-like changes.[42] A central scar, clinically and histologically similar to a recurrent/persistent nevus, may also become noticeable and probably is a sequel to partial involution of the nevus or to folliculitis. The lack of cytologic atypia and mitoses help differentiate these nevi from a regressing melanoma.[43] Basal cell carcinoma has also been reported to occur in collision with a melanocytic nevus.[44,45]

Pitfalls
Congenital melanocytic nevi

1. The lentiginous melanocytic hyperplasia often seen in CMN may lead to an incorrect diagnosis of an atypical or dysplastic nevus
2. The variation in size and shape of junctional nests together with pagetoid spread of melanocytes may be misinterpreted as melanoma in situ
3. Proliferative nodules within CMN may be misdiagnosed as melanoma developing within the nevus
4. The junctional component of a recurrent/persistent congenital melanocytic nevus may be mistaken for melanoma in situ

SUMMARY

CMN are present at birth or appear shortly thereafter and present with characteristic histopathologic features, such as symmetry, good circumscription, uniform nests in the epidermis equidistant from each other, nests of melanocytes and individual melanocytes in the dermis that mature with their descent, wrapping of nevus cells around vessels and adnexal structures, and splaying of melanocytes in-between collagen bundles. There are several histologic variants of CMN. Congenital features may also be observed in biopsies of melanocytic nevi in adults with no clear history of congenital onset. Pathologists should be aware of important histologic pitfalls when making the diagnosis of a congenital melanocytic nevus, such as lentiginous melanocytic hyperplasia, pagetoid spread, and proliferative nodules, among others. CMN should be differentiated from dysplastic nevi with congenital pattern and nevoid melanoma.

REFERENCES

1. Ingordo V, Gentile C, Iannazzone SS, et al. Congenital melanocytic nevus: an epidemiologic study in Italy. Dermatology 2007;214(3):227–30.
2. Haupt HM, Stern JB. Pagetoid melanocytosis. Histologic features in benign and malignant lesions. Am J Surg Pathol 1995;19(7):792–7.
3. Castilla EE, da Graca Dutra M, Orioli-Parreiras IM. Epidemiology of congenital pigmented naevi: I. Incidence rates and relative frequencies. Br J Dermatol 1981;104(3):307–15.
4. Swerdlow AJ, English JS, Qiao Z. The risk of melanoma in patients with congenital nevi: a cohort study. J Am Acad Dermatol 1995;32(4):595–9.
5. Sahin S, Levin L, Kopf AW, et al. Risk of melanoma in medium-sized congenital melanocytic nevi: a follow-up study. J Am Acad Dermatol 1998;39(3):428–33.
6. Lorentzen M, Pers M, Bretteville-Jensen G. The incidence of malignant transformation in giant pigmented nevi. Scand J Plast Reconstr Surg 1977;11(2):163–7.
7. DeDavid M, Orlow SJ, Provost N, et al. A study of large congenital melanocytic nevi and associated malignant melanomas: review of cases in the New York University Registry and the world literature. J Am Acad Dermatol 1997;36(3 Pt 1):409–16.
8. Quaedvlieg PJ, Frank J, Vermeulen AH, et al. Giant ceribriform intradermal nevus on the back of a newborn. Pediatr Dermatol 2008;25(1):43–6.
9. Barnhill RL, Fleischli M. Histologic features of congenital melanocytic nevi in infants 1 year of age or younger. J Am Acad Dermatol 1995;33(5 Pt 1):780–5.
10. Mark GJ, Mihm MC, Liteplo MG, et al. Congenital melanocytic nevi of the small and garment type. Clinical, histologic, and ultrastructural studies. Hum Pathol 1973;4(3):395–418.
11. Jensen SL, Radfar A, Bhawan J. Mitoses in conventional melanocytic nevi. J Cutan Pathol 2007;34(9):713–5.
12. Rhodes AR, Silverman RA, Harrist TJ, et al. A histologic comparison of congenital and acquired nevomelanocytic nevi. Arch Dermatol 1985;121(10):1266–73.
13. Solomon L, Eng AM, Bene M, et al. Giant congenital neuroid melanocytic nevus. Arch Dermatol 1980;116(3):318–20.
14. Stefanaki C, Stefanaki K, Antoniou C, et al. Cell cycle and apoptosis regulators in Spitz nevi: comparison with melanomas and common nevi. J Am Acad Dermatol 2007;56(5):815–24.
15. Bastian BC, Olshen AB, LeBoit PE, et al. Classifying melanocytic tumors based on DNA copy number changes. Am J Pathol 2003;163(5):1765–70.

16. Bastian BC, Xiong J, Frieden IJ, et al. Genetic changes in neoplasms arising in congenital melanocytic nevi: differences between nodular proliferations and melanomas. Am J Pathol 2002;161(4):1163–9.
17. Illig L, Weidner F, Hundeiker M, et al. Congenital nevi less than or equal to 10 cm as precursors to melanoma. 52 cases, a review, and a new conception. Arch Dermatol 1985;121(10):1274–81.
18. Hendrickson MR, Ross JC. Neoplasms arising in congenital giant nevi: morphologic study of seven cases and a review of the literature. Am J Surg Pathol 1981; 5(2):109–35.
19. Mancianti ML, Clark WH, Hayes FA, et al. Malignant melanoma simulants arising in congenital melanocytic nevi do not show experimental evidence for a malignant phenotype. Am J Pathol 1990;136(4):817–29.
20. Toussaint S, Kamino H. Dysplastic changes in different types of melanocytic nevi. A unifying concept. J Cutan Pathol 1999;26(2):84–90.
21. Boyd AS, Rapini RP. Acral melanocytic neoplasms: a histologic analysis of 158 lesions. J Am Acad Dermatol 1994;31(5 Pt 1):740–5.
22. Clemente C, Zurrida S, Bartoli C, et al. Acral-lentiginous naevus of plantar skin. Histopathology 1995;27(6):549–55.
23. Xu X, Bellucci KS, Elenitsas R, et al. Cellular nodules in congenital pattern nevi. J Cutan Pathol 2004;31(2):153–9.
24. Murphy MJ, Jen M, Chang MW, et al. Molecular diagnosis of a benign proliferative nodule developing in a congenital melanocytic nevus in a 3-month-old infant. J Am Acad Dermatol 2008;59(3):518–23.
25. Arrese Estrada J, Pierard-Franchimont C, Pierard GE. Histogenesis of recurrent nevus. Am J Dermatopathol 1990;12(4):370–2.
26. Harvell JD, Bastian BC, LeBoit PE. Persistent (recurrent) Spitz nevi: a histopathologic, immunohistochemical, and molecular pathologic study of 22 cases. Am J Surg Pathol 2002;26(5):654–61.
27. Hoang MP, Prieto VG, Burchette JL, et al. Recurrent melanocytic nevus: a histologic and immunohistochemical evaluation. J Cutan Pathol 2001;28(8): 400–6.
28. Sexton M, Sexton CW. Recurrent pigmented melanocytic nevus. A benign lesion, not to be mistaken for malignant melanoma. Arch Pathol Lab Med 1991;115(2): 122–6.
29. Park HK, Leonard DD, Arrington JH 3rd, et al. Recurrent melanocytic nevi: clinical and histologic review of 175 cases. J Am Acad Dermatol 1987;17(2 Pt 1):285–92.
30. Schaffer JV. Pigmented lesions in children: when to worry. Curr Opin Pediatr 2007;19(4):430–40.
31. Rhodes AR, Melski JW. Small congenital nevocellular nevi and the risk of cutaneous melanoma. J Pediatr 1982;100(2):219–24.
32. Tannous ZS, Mihm MC Jr, Sober AJ, et al. Congenital melanocytic nevi: clinical and histopathologic features, risk of melanoma, and clinical management. J Am Acad Dermatol 2005;52(2):197–203.
33. Swerdlow AJ, Green A. Melanocytic naevi and melanoma: an epidemiological perspective. Br J Dermatol 1987;117(2):137–46.
34. Elder DE, Elenitsas R, Murphy GF, et al. Benign pigmented lesions and malignant melanoma. In: Lever WF, Elder DE, editors. Lever's histopathology of the skin. 9th edition. Philadelphia: Lippincott Williams & Wilkins; 2005. p. 715–803.
35. Bouffard D, Barnhill RL, Mihm MC, et al. Very late metastasis (27 years) of cutaneous malignant melanoma arising in a halo giant congenital nevus. Dermatology 1994;189(2):162–6.

36. Betti R, Inselvini E, Palvarini M, et al. Agminate and plaque-type blue nevus combined with lentigo, associated with follicular cyst and eccrine changes: a variant of speckled lentiginous nevus. Dermatology 1997;195(4):387–90.
37. Requena L, Ambrojo P, Sanchez Yus E. Trichilemmal cyst under a compound melanocytic nevus. J Cutan Pathol 1990;17(3):185–8.
38. Tomasini C, Broganelli P, Pippione M. Targetoid hemosiderotic nevus. A trauma-induced simulator of malignant melanoma. Dermatology 2005;210(3):200–5.
39. Schaefer JT, Nuovo GJ, Yen BT, et al. Prominent eosinophilic intranuclear inclusions in melanocytes of a melanocytic nevus: the aftermath of an infection with molluscum contagiosum? A case report. J Cutan Pathol 2008;35(8):782–8.
40. Hahm GK, McMahon JT, Nuovo GJ, et al. Eosinophilic intranuclear inclusion bodies in a melanocytic nevus. Cutis 2002;69(3):223–6.
41. King R, Googe PB, Page RN, et al. Melanocytic lesions associated with dermatofibromas: a spectrum of lesions ranging from junctional nevus to malignant melanoma in situ. Mod Pathol 2005;18(8):1043–7.
42. Horenstein MG, Prieto VG, Burchette JL Jr, et al. Keratotic melanocytic nevus: a clinicopathologic and immunohistochemical study. J Cutan Pathol 2000;27(7):344–50.
43. Fabrizi G, Pennacchia I, Pagliarello C, et al. Sclerosing nevus with pseudomelanomatous features. J Cutan Pathol 2008;35(11):995–1002.
44. de Giorgi V, Massi D, Sestini S, et al. Cutaneous collision tumour (melanocytic naevus, basal cell carcinoma, seborrhoeic keratosis): a clinical, dermoscopic and pathological case report. Br J Dermatol 2005;152(4):787–90.
45. Taira JW, Flaming JA, Weigand DA. Basal cell carcinoma and melanocytic nevus in the same lesion. Cutis 1992;49(1):40–2.

Acral Lentiginous Melanoma

Melissa Peck Piliang, MD

KEYWORDS

• Melanoma • Acral • Palms • Soles • Nevi

OVERVIEW: ACRAL LENTIGINOUS MELANOMA

Acral lentiginous melanoma (ALM), the least common of the four major subtypes of cutaneous malignant melanoma, was first described by Reed[1] in 1976. As the name suggests, ALM occurs on acral skin, namely the palms, soles, and nails. It is an uncommon cutaneous tumor that occurs in all races at the same rate.[2] In persons with lighter skin types, who have an overall higher incidence of melanoma in general, ALM is the least common of the four major subtypes, accounting for 4% to 10% of all melanoma diagnoses whereas it is the most common subtype in darker skin types (Asians, Middle Easterners, and Africans), who have a lower overall incidence of melanoma.[3] This reflects the lower incidence of melanomas elsewhere on the body in the more pigmented skin types. Patients with ALM have a poor prognosis, in part because they present with more advanced disease.[4–6]

Although the pathogenesis of ALM remains unknown, it has been theorized that the more intense and chronic trauma experienced in acral locations may be a predisposing factor.

Key Features
Acral lentiginous melanoma

1. Asymmetric and poorly circumscribed
2. Primarily lentiginous growth of single melanocytes at the dermoepidermal junction over a nested or pagetoid growth pattern
3. Cytologic atypia
4. Dermal component that is spindle cell with desmoplastic stroma
5. Deep dermal mitoses
6. Lack of maturation

A version of this article was previously published in *Surgical Pathology Clinics* 2:3.
Department of Dermatology and Department of Anatomic Pathology, Cleveland Clinic, Cleveland Clinic Foundation, 9500 Euclid Avenue – A61, Cleveland, OH 44195, USA
E-mail address: pilianm@ccf.org

Clin Lab Med 31 (2011) 281–288
doi:10.1016/j.cll.2011.03.005 **labmed.theclinics.com**
0272-2712/11/$ – see front matter

ALM has a unique patient profile among subtypes of melanoma. In comparison to the other frequent melanoma variants, ALM patients have key demographic and lifestyle differences to distinguish ALM from other melanoma subtypes: it occurs in an older patient population, and is associated with a lower number of common and atypical nevi, a lower incidence of familial melanoma, and a lower incidence of sunburn but a higher personal and family history of noncutaneous cancers.[7,8]

ALM must be distinguished from acral lentiginous nevi, which can display well-described site-related atypia, fibrohistiocytic lesions, and poorly differentiated carcinoma.

GROSS PATHOLOGY

Like many entities in dermatopathology, the gross examination is best described in vivo and, therefore, must rely on clinician skill and knowledge. ALMs present on the palms and soles as pigmented macules or papules with variegated pigment and irregular borders. More advanced tumors present as large, exophytic, friable nodules. Often, ALM is darkly pigmented and may appear blue-black, although amelanotic lesions occur as red-pink macules or nodules. In contrast, acral lentiginous nevi are smaller, light-brown, uniform macules with well-circumscribed borders. Lesions of ALM may have been present for years, although some patients report recently noticing a lesion, frequently after trauma to the foot or due to associated symptoms. Lesions may have been previously clinically diagnosed as warts, pyogenic granulomas, or other vascular tumors, hematomas, or ulcers. Symptoms associated with ALM include pain, bleeding, and itching. Subungual ALM presents as pigmented streaks (melanonychia striata) in the nail plate that extend as dark pigmentation onto the proximal or lateral nail fold (Hutchinson's sign).

MICROSCOPIC FEATURES

Histology

The histologic findings of ALM are characterized by an asymmetric, poorly circumscribed proliferation of continuous single melanocytes at the dermoepidermal junction (**Figs. 1** and **2**). Single melanocytes predominate over nests (see **Fig. 1**). The melanocytes are hyperchromatic with enlarged nuclei; overt pleomorphism, however, is uncommon. The intraepidermal melanocytes often have dendritic cytoplasmic processes and are surrounded by a clear halo imparting a somewhat stellate appearance to the tumor cells. This morphology can be a clue to the diagnosis. Development of nests is seen later in the evolution of the tumor, with elongated nests arranged parallel to the epidermis. Similarly, prominent pagetoid spread tends to be a late feature in ALM. As expected in an acral site, the epidermis is hyperplastic with

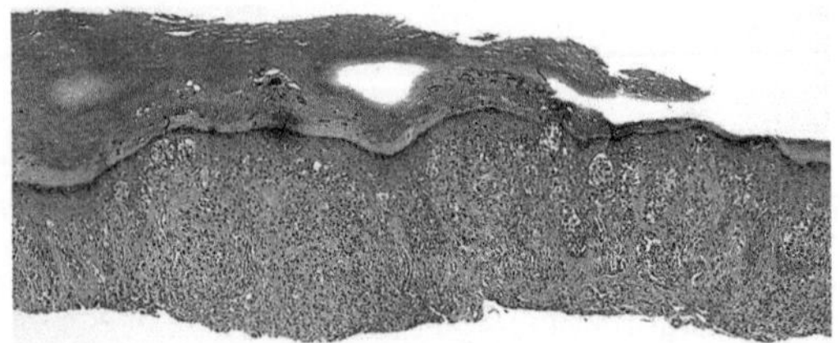

Fig. 1. Acral lentiginous melanoma: low-power images showing a poorly circumscribed proliferation of atypical melanocytes in the epidermis and dermis with marked lentinginous and pagetoid spread of individual melanocytes.

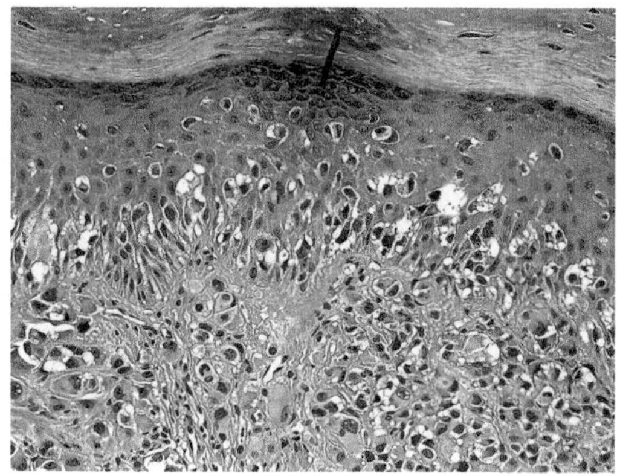

Fig. 2. Acral lentiginous melanoma: medium-power image showing large atypical single melanocytes at all levels of epidermis and in the dermis without maturation of dermal component.

elongated rete and overlying compact orthokeratotic stratum corneum, which may be heavily pigmented. The dermal component, if present, is often spindle-shaped with a desmoplastic stroma and lacks maturation (**Fig. 3**). The presence of deep dermal mitoses is a clue to the diagnosis of ALM. ALM frequently has an associated lymphocytic infiltrate in the underlying dermis, and the presence of inflammation can be a clue to the diagnosis. Another important feature of ALM is frequent skip areas within the tumor. As a result, clinically pigmented parts of the lesion may be devoid of melanocytes in small biopsy specimens.

Immunohistochemistry

Immunohistochemistry can be helpful in equivocal or unusual cases but is most often not necessary and, in some cases, may actually add to diagnostic dilemma. S-100 protein is a sensitive but nonspecific marker with a positivity rate of greater than 95% in ALM, comparable to nonacral melanomas.[9] HMB-45, which stains premelanosome glycoprotein, may be helpful in cases of ALM. In a study by Kim and colleagues,[9]

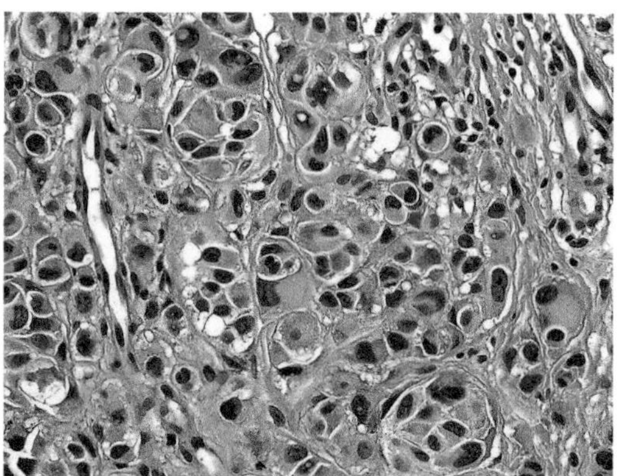

Fig. 3. Acral lentiginous melanoma: high-power image of the dermal melanocytes showing large, atypical nuclei.

16 of 20 (80%) cases of ALM stained with HMB-45. The HMB-45–negative cases were all amelanotic tumors, although three of seven amelanotic cases were positive for HMB-45.

Ki-67 antibody, a proliferative marker, can be helpful to assess the mitotic activity of the dermal component; however, Ki-67 should be interpreted with caution, because lymphocytes within an associated lymphocytic infiltrate also are highlighted. Furthermore, not all cases of ALM have a high nuclear labeling index in the dermal component. Interpretation, therefore, is highly dependent on the histologic context.

Infrequently, ALM stains positive for epithelial markers. Generally, in these cases, the melanocytes stain with one or more of the melanocytic markers also. Therefore, in cases where it is necessary to rule out a poorly differentiated carcinoma, S-100 and HMB-45 positivity in the tumor cells, despite focal epithelial marker positivity, is helpful.[9]

DIFFERENTIAL DIAGNOSIS OF ACRAL LENTIGINOUS MELANOMA

ALM can be difficult to distinguish from acral lentiginous nevi. Acral lentiginous nevi can have histologic features that overlap significantly with ALM. Because of this, overdiagnosis and underdiagnosis of melanoma is a risk in the interpretation of melanocytic lesions from this anatomic location.[10] Benign acral nevi are usually symmetric and composed mostly of nested melanocytes, although some lentiginous growth of single melanocytes is acceptable.

The low-power image is often helpful displaying a symmetric, primarily nested growth pattern with dermal skip areas and syringotropism (**Fig. 4**). Symmetry and circumscription (lateral borders ending in nests rather than single melanocytes) may be difficult to assess if the lesion is not completely removed.

Differential Diagnosis
Acral lentiginous melanoma

Acral lentiginous nevus

- Significant overlap of histologic features of benign acral nevi with ALM
- Benign acral nevi
- Usually symmetric
- Composed mostly of nested melanocytes, with some lentiginous growth of single melanocytes acceptable
- Low-power image helpful in displaying a symmetric, primarily nested growth pattern with dermal skip areas and syringotropism
- Circumscription, with lateral borders ending in nests rather than single melanocytes
- Nests, when present, are often large and confluent in ALM
- Upward migration of melanocytes is more orderly, may be nested and, usually centrally located

Atypical melanocytic nevus

Fibrohistiocytic tumor

Poorly differentiated carcinoma

- Panel of epithelial markers and melanocytic markers needed to exclude a poorly differentiated carcinoma

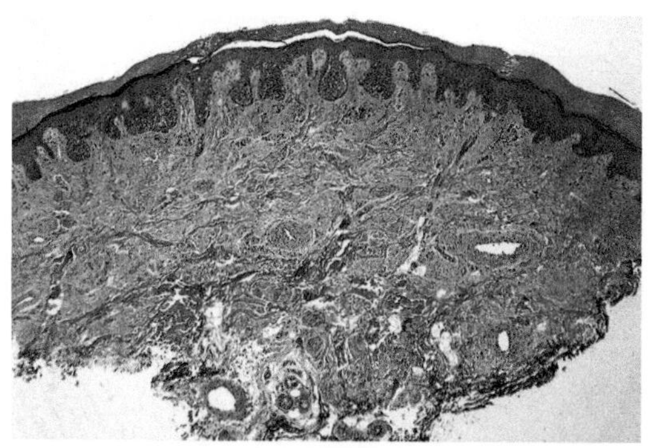

Fig. 4. Acral lentiginous nevus: low-power image showing a well-circumscribed melanocytic proliferation of primarily nested melanocytes at the dermoepidermal junction with low-level pagetoid spread.

The histologic features of the epidermal component are critical in differentiating benign acral lentiginous nevi from ALM.[6] Although lentiginous growth can be seen in acral nevi, the growth pattern is predominantly small nests admixed with single melanocytes at the dermoepidermal junction (**Figs. 4** and **5**). In contrast, melanoma at acral sites exhibits a marked predominance of lentiginous single melanocytes at the lower levels of the epidermis over nests. Nests, when present, are often large and confluent in ALM.

The presence of upward migration of melanocytes into the overlying epidermis of acral nevi, possibly related to chronic trauma at acral sites,[10] is a pitfall that can lead to misdiagnosis as ALM. The upward migration of melanocytes, however, is more orderly, may be nested, and, importantly, is usually centrally located (**Fig. 6**).[11] Pagetoid spread in ALM, when present, is haphazard and not restricted to the central portion of the lesion. Cytologic atypia in the junctional component, as discussed previously, help distinguish ALM from acral nevi.[11]

If present, the dermal component of acral nevi shows maturation, bland cytology, and no mitotic or proliferative activity. An inflammatory infiltrate is usually lacking in acral nevi. The dermal component of ALM often has a spindle cell morphology and dermal mitotic activity and is frequently accompanied by a lymphocytic infiltrate.

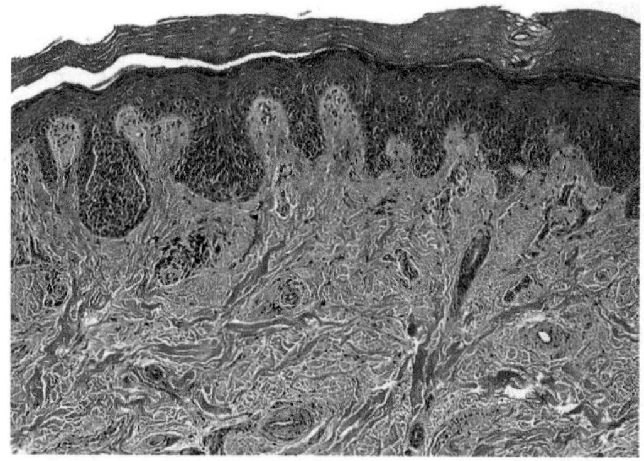

Fig. 5. Acral lentiginous nevus: medium-power image showing primarily nested melanocytes at the dermoepidermal junction with low-level pagetoid spread.

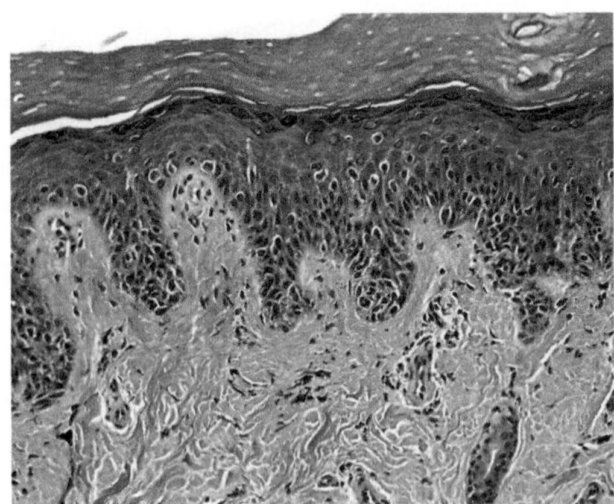

Fig. 6. Acral lentiginous nevus: high-power image showing nested and single melanocytes without cytologic atypia.

In selected cases, immunohistochemistry can be helpful in distinguishing ALM from an acral nevus. Immunohistochemical stains for HMB-45 usually highlight both the junctional and dermal component of ALM. In acral nevi, HMB-45 usually highlights only the junctional component; staining in the dermal component is usually absent or limited. Ki-67 can be helpful to evaluate for proliferative activity of the dermal component when there is not significant lymphocytic inflammation. Although immunohistochemistry can be helpful to support a histologic diagnosis in melanocytic lesions, there is great variability in staining, and the diagnosis of benign acral nevus or acral melanoma should not be based on immunohistochemistry alone.

Occasionally, a poorly differentiated carcinoma is in the histologic differential diagnosis for acral lesions. A panel of epithelial markers (eg, epithelial membrane antigen and cytokeratins AE1/3 and CAM5.2) and melanocytic markers (S-100, Melan-A, and HMB-45) is needed to exclude a poorly differentiated carcinoma.[9] ALMs can infrequently show focal staining with one or more epithelial markers. In this instance, positivity to one of more of the melanocytic markers is important to correctly diagnose the melanoma.

PROGNOSIS OF ACRAL LENTIGINOUS MELANOMA

ALM has a worse prognosis than the other subtypes of melanoma, even when controlling for tumor thickness. There are several reasons for this phenomenon, which include the inherent biologic behavior of acral melanoma, difficulty in identifying and diagnosing these tumors, and overall health of the affected patients, who tend to be older than other patients with melanoma.

The key factor in survival for all melanomas is stage and tumor thickness at diagnosis. Early diagnosis of melanoma, when tumors are thinner, portends a better overall survival.[3,6,12] The earlier the melanoma is diagnosed, the better the prognosis. For many reasons, ALM is diagnosed at a more advanced stage than other melanomas. These include occurrences in areas that are not accessible to casual observation, areas that have limited sun exposure, and sites that are more difficult to biopsy.

In addition, ALM may mimic other benign entities thus delaying diagnosis or leading to incorrect therapies. The average age of patients diagnosed with ALM is significantly older than of those who have melanomas, portending a poorer prognosis.

Pitfalls
Acral lentiginous melanoma

! ALM may show weak or focal positivity for epithelial markers (EMA and CAM 5.2). Melanocytic markers (S-100, HMB-45, and Melan-A) should be positive.

! Care should be taken with benign-appearing lesions that are incompletely excised or with a lentiginous component trailing to the biopsy margin.

! The presence of extensive centrally located pagetoid spread without other atypical features should not lead to the diagnosis of ALM. Acral nevi can show extensive pagetoid spread.

! ALMs frequently have skip areas devoid of the melanocytic proliferation. If a clinician suspects melanoma but biopsy findings are negative or equivocal, additional biopsies should be performed.

The histologic prognostic indicators for melanoma include Breslow thickness, Clark level, ulceration, dermal mitoses, and evidence of intravascular or neural involvement. Recent reports of large cohorts of patients with ALM have shown that male gender and clinical amelanosis are associated with a greater Breslow thickness and worse prognosis.[3,4] Cultural and socioeconomic factors may also play a role; Hispanic whites and Asian/Pacific Islanders present at more advanced stage than non-Hispanics, resulting in a poorer prognosis.[3] Overall survival rate among all racial groups do not show statistically significant variation when controlled for Breslow thickness and tumor stage at diagnosis.[3]

SUMMARY

ALM is an uncommon form of cutaneous malignant melanoma that occurs at equal incidence in all races and is not correlated to lifetime sun exposure or sunburns. Key histologic findings are a poorly circumscribed, asymmetric lentiginous proliferation of atypical single melanocytes at the dermoepidermal junction. When a dermal component is present, deep dermal mitoses, spindle cell morphology with a desmoplastic stroma, and lack of maturation are suggestive of ALM over a benign nevus. Immunohistochemical markers have limited use in confirming melanocytic derivation and ruling out poorly differentiated carcinoma. ALM is diagnosed in older patients and at a more advanced stage than other melanomas, thus leading to a worse prognosis.

REFERENCES

1. Reed RJ. Acral lentiginous melanoma. In: Hartman W, Kay S, Reed RJ, editors. New concepts in surgical pathology of the skin. New York: Wiley; 1976. p. 89–90.
2. Bristow IR, Acland K. Acral lentiginous melanoma of the foot and ankle: a case series and review of the literature. J Foot Ankle Res 2008;1:11.
3. Bradford PT, Goldstein AM, McMaster ML, et al. Acral lentiginous melanoma incidence and survival patterns in the United States, 1986–2005. Arch Dermatol 2009;145(4):427–34.
4. Phan A, Touzet S, Dalle S, et al. Acral lentiginous melanoma: a clincoprognostic study of 126 cases. Br J Dermatol 2006;155:561–9.
5. Kogushi-Nishi H, Kawasaki TK, Ishihara T, et al. The prevalence of melanocytic nevi on the soles in the Japanese population. J Am Acad Dermatol 2009;60:767–71.
6. Phan A, Touzet S, Dalle S, et al. Acral lentiginous melanoma: histopathological prognostic features of 121 cases. Br J Dermatol 2007;157(2):311–8.

7. Soudry E, Gutman H, Feinmesser M, et al. "Gloves-and-socks" melanoma: does histology make a difference. Dermatol Surg 2008;34:1372–8.
8. Nagore E, Pereda C, Botella-Estrada R, et al. Acral lentiginous melanoma presents distinct clinical profile with high cancer susceptibility. Cancer Causes Control 2009;20:115–9.
9. Kim YC, Lee MG, Choe SW, et al. Acral lentiginous melanoma: an immunohistochemical study of 20 cases. Int J Dermatol 2003;42:123–9.
10. Hosler GA, Moresi JM, Barrett TL. Nevi with site-related atypia: a review of melanocytic nevi with atypical histologic features based on anatomic site. J Cutan Pathol 2008;35:889–98.
11. Tan K, Moncrieff M, Thompson JF, et al. Subungual melanoma a study of 124 cases highlighting features of early lesions, potential pitfalls in diagnosis, and guidelines for histologic reporting. Am J Surg Pathol 2007;31(12):1902–12.
12. Kwon H, Lee JH, Cho KH. Acral lentiginous melanoma in situ: a study of nine cases. Am J Dermatopathol 2004;26:285–9.

Melanoma Margin Assessment

Martin J. Trotter, MD, PhD, FRCPC

KEYWORDS

• Margin assessment • Melanoma in situ • Zentigo maligna
• Frozen sections • Immunohistochemistry

OVERVIEW: MARGIN ASSESSMENT

Primary cutaneous melanoma is treated by excisional surgery. The pathologist is responsible for assessment of the excised tissue margins and must determine whether the margins are free of melanoma. Careful interpretation of specimen margins is a crucial component of the pathologic reporting of cutaneous melanoma.[1]

METHODS OF MARGIN ASSESSMENT

Several methods may be used to assess the margins of cutaneous melanoma excision specimens (**Table 1**).[2–4] Conventional vertical sections, perpendicular to the skin surface, may be transverse, bread-loafing the specimen; longitudinal, usually as part of a cross technique; or peripheral (perimeter or en face sections). Horizontal sections may be used to sample the deep surgical margin. Mohs micrographic surgery (MMS) employs oblique sections that simultaneously sample peripheral and deep margins.[5]

Transverse (bread-loaf) Vertical Sections

Conventional vertical sections, obtained perpendicular to the resection margin, allow examination of the entire spectrum of histology within the lesion and facilitate identification of the transition between invasive melanoma, melanoma in situ, atypical melanocytic hyperplasia, and normal skin (**Fig. 1**).[6] Also, measurement of the distance from the tumor to the margin can be performed. However, bread-loaf sections are a form of step sections, and therefore allow the histologic examination of only a small percentage of the actual specimen margin. Bread-loafing has a low sensitivity for detecting margins positive for melanoma in situ and it has been predicted that "bread-loafing at 1-, 2-, 4-, and 10-mm intervals would have only a 58%, 37%, 19%, and 7% chance of detecting a positive margin" given an average linear extent

A version of this article was previously published in *Surgical Pathology Clinics* 2:3.
Department of Pathology and Laboratory Medicine, University of Calgary, Calgary Laboratory Services, 9-3535 Research Road NW, Calgary, Alberta, Canada T2L 2K8
E-mail address: martin.trotter@cls.ab.ca

Clin Lab Med 31 (2011) 289–300
doi:10.1016/j.cll.2011.03.006 labmed.theclinics.com
0272-2712/11/$ – see front matter

Table 1
Methods of margin assessment

Margin Assessment	Advantages	Disadvantages
Vertical, transverse sections	Can assess the entire spectrum of melanoma pathology from center to margin of specimen Can measure the distance of the tumor from the surgical margin	Sample only a small percentage of the surgical margin
Vertical, peripheral (en face) sections	Sample close to 100% of the surgical margin	Not useful for melanoma with a discontinuous growth pattern May be difficult to obtain from curved or irregularly shaped specimens May be difficult to embed or section resulting in incomplete sampling of epidermal margin
Oblique sections (Mohs)	Sample close to 100% of the surgical margin, including the deep margin	Frozen sections commonly used, with decreased ability to diagnose subtle lesions May be difficult to embed or section resulting in incomplete sampling of epidermal margin

of melanoma at the surgical margin of 1.4 mm.[6] To sample close to 100% of the peripheral margin step sections at intervals of 0.1 mm would be required.

En Face Vertical Sections

En face vertical sections sample close to 100% of the surgical margin, although they may be difficult to obtain from curved or irregularly shaped melanoma excision specimens (**Fig. 2**). These margins must be embedded and cut correctly, using ink to identify the true surgical margin, and ensuring complete sections are available for

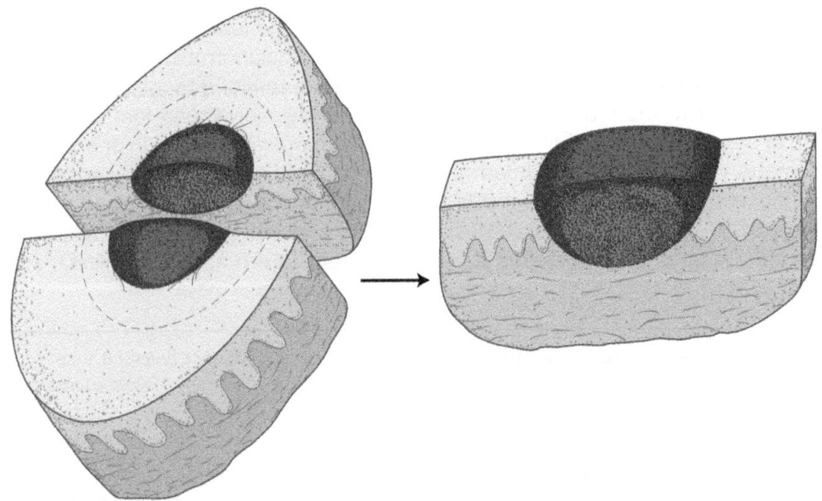

Fig. 1. Transverse (bread-loaf) vertical sections through the center of the excision specimen.

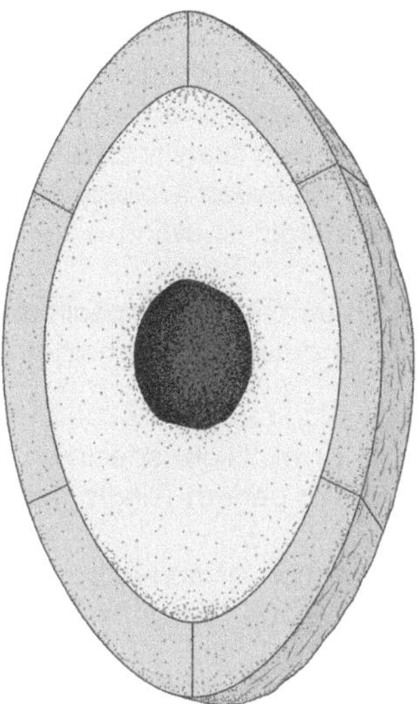

Fig. 2. En face vertical sections from the perimeter of the excision specimen.

assessment. En face sections are not appropriate for melanomas with a noncontinuous growth pattern (see later discussion).

En Face Oblique Sections

En face oblique sections (eg, MMS) also sample, in addition to 100% of the peripheral margin, the deep specimen margin. Embedding and sectioning of specimens hold the same challenges as vertical en face sections. When frozen sections are used, the quality of the histology is diminished compared with formalin-fixed, paraffin-embedded sections, and interpretation may be difficult for subtle lesions.

Choice of sectioning method depends on anatomic location and the growth pattern of the melanoma. Studies suggest that lentigo maligna (LM) and acral lentiginous pattern melanomas demonstrate uninterrupted, contiguous spread into the periphery at the epidermal-dermal junction, but superficial spreading and nodular pattern melanomas show noncontinuous, subclinical spread.[7] Thus, methods that sample a thin strip of the entire peripheral margin (en face or Mohs techniques) are most suitable for lentigo maligna melanoma (LMM) or acral lentiginous melanoma. These techniques are probably not appropriate for superficial spreading melanoma and nodular melanoma.

MARGIN ASSESSMENT FOR MELANOMA ON SUN-DAMAGED SKIN

There is considerably controversy regarding how best to evaluate excision margins for melanoma arising in sun-damaged skin. Margin assessment for these melanomas is problematic because lesions are often clinically ill defined and the histology of lentigo maligna (in situ melanoma) overlaps considerably with changes seen in normal skin with chronic actinic damage. Invasive components can also have bland morphology mimicking benign nevi or scar. Cosmetic and functional considerations are of great importance because most of these lesions arise in the head and neck region. Two main issues require discussion: How do we define a positive margin and what is the best method for margin evaluation?

Definition of a Positive Surgical Margin

Dermatopathologists have not agreed upon a uniform definition of a positive margin for LM. LM and melanocytic hyperplasia on chronically sun-damaged skin are related to cumulative sun exposure and likely form part of a continuum.[8] Thus, there is considerable histologic overlap between a biologically important positive margin containing LM and a negative margin showing solar melanocytic hyperplasia or solar lentigo.

Examination of the original excision, or debulk, specimen and of control sun-exposed skin specimens may be helpful in determining whether a LM margin is involved by tumor:

- Examination of the debulk, or excision, specimen allows determination of the predominant melanoma in situ pattern (single cell, nested, pigmentation, and so forth).
- Examination of a control section of sun-exposed skin (eg, superficial shave biopsy from opposite cheek) allows recognition of the background level of melanocytic hyperplasia.[9]

In situ melanoma, lentigo maligna pattern

The following histologic features indicate the presence of LM in an excision margin, although no single feature is specific (**Fig. 3**).[8,10–13]

- Nests of melanocytes
- Markedly increased numbers of melanocytes in the epidermis (eg, >25 melanocytes per 0.5 mm of basal layer)
- Pagetoid spread
- Contiguous melanocytes in basal epidermis
- Significant cytologic atypia
- Multinucleated melanocytes (starburst cells)[14]
- Significant adnexal involvement
- Uneven pigmentation
- Melanophages
- Lymphocytic infiltrate.

Although the center of a LM lesion may exhibit most of the above features, the periphery is often poorly defined clinically and histologically, and appearances overlap with normal sun-exposed skin, especially if sun-induced melanocytic hyperplasia is present. Nesting of melanocytes, especially if nests are large, is suggestive of

Key Features
Histologic features of melanoma in situ on sun-damaged skin

1. Intraepidermal pagetoid spread
2. Junctional or intraepidermal nests of melanocytes
3. Groups of greater than or equal to three contiguous melanocytes in basal epidermis
4. Markedly increased number of single melanocytes in basal epidermis (eg, 50 melanocytes per 1.0 mm)
5. Marked cytologic atypia, including multinucleate melanocytes (starburst cells)
6. Significant adnexal involvement

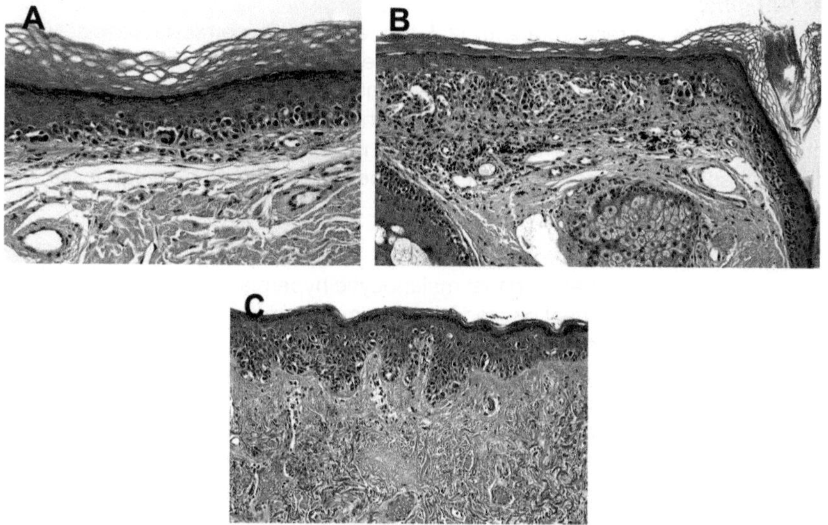

Fig. 3. Melanoma in situ on sun-damaged skin showing contiguous atypical melanocytes in basal epidermis (*A*). Nests of atypical melanocytes (*B*) and pagetoid spread (*C*).

melanoma. Nested pattern LM often has melanocyte nests similar to those seen in dysplastic nevus[15] or pigmented spindle cell nevus.[8]

Solar melanocytic hyperplasia

The degree of melanocytic hyperplasia observed in chronically sun-exposed skin may be quite striking (**Fig. 4**). In several studies of sun-exposed, uninvolved skin adjacent to melanoma or nonmelanoma skin cancers the mean number of melanocytes was 3.9 to 15.6 per 0.5 mm of epidermis (typical high-power field).[11–13,16] Melanocyte confluence, formation of small nests, adnexal extension, and nuclear atypia have all been observed. Thus, there is considerable histologic overlap between solar melanocytic hyperplasia and atypical melanocytic hyperplasia at the margins of in situ melanoma, LM pattern.

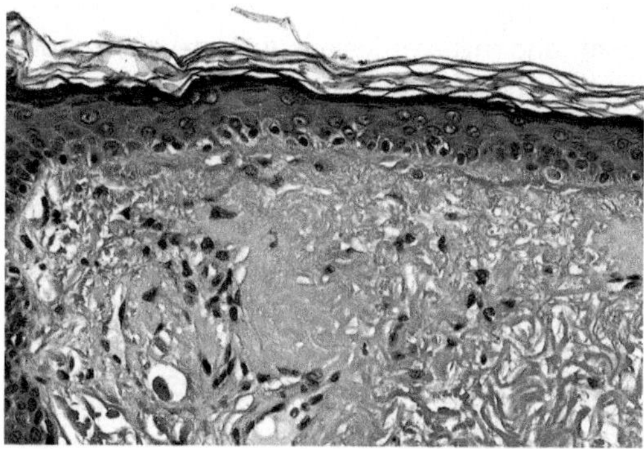

Fig. 4. Melanocytic hyperplasia (solar melanocytosis) in nonlesional (clinically nonpigmented) sun-damaged skin.

Solar lentigines
Solar lentigines of the face frequently lack the rete ridge hyperplasia classically associated with lentigines from other anatomic sites.[17] These lentigines have increased melanocytes (mean 2.1-fold increase over normal sun-exposed facial skin) and increased epidermal melanin (2.2-fold higher than baseline sun-exposed facial skin). Contiguous lesions of solar lentigo are present in 23% of LM excision specimens[18,19] and the flat solar lentigo of facial skin[17] must be recognized as a benign lesion in LM excision margin assessment.

Field effect
Previously some authors believed that melanocytic hyperplasia adjacent to melanoma was secondary to a field effect caused by the primary tumor.[20] However, other studies suggest that the field change effect in epidermal melanocytes adjacent to melanoma is the result of chronic sun exposure alone.[16,21] Genetic evidence for a field effect has been obtained in acral melanoma[22,23] and a recent study of normal sun-exposed skin adjacent to skin cancer showed that solar melanocytic hyperplasia with atypical features (contiguous melanocytes, atypical melanocytes, follicular extension) was more commonly observed in specimens from subjects who had melanoma than in specimens from subjects who had nonmelanoma skin cancer.[13]

Melanocytic hyperplasia secondary to previous biopsy
Melanocytic hyperplasia, presumably occurring as a reactive phenomenon to a previous surgical procedure, is well described.[24,25] In the study by Duve and colleagues,[25] 8% of skin re-excision specimens showed significant melanocytic hyperplasia (almost all of these were specimens from sun-exposed skin of the face and neck), but this hyperplasia was well circumscribed and confined to the epidermis above the scar. If scar is present in the margins for lentigo maligna, then this pattern of intraepidermal melanocytic hyperplasia should be considered.

Lichenoid reactions
Lichenoid reactions, especially those with pseudonest formation, complicate the interpretation of LM margins.[26] Pseudonests[27] closely mimic nesting in LM, including having occasional Melan-A positivity. Lichenoid reactions in dark-skinned individuals can closely mimic LM histologically.

Invasive melanoma
Invasive melanoma is rarely seen at the peripheral margins of melanoma excisions from sun-damaged skin. These margins usually only contain in situ melanoma. Nevertheless, two obvious pitfalls should be considered: desmoplastic melanoma (mimicking biopsy scar) and invasive lesions with nevoid morphology. The latter is not uncommon in lentigo maligna melanoma, where the invasive component may be extremely subtle, bland, and nevoid. Any dermal component observed in a melanoma margin should be considered melanoma until proven otherwise. Usually, careful histologic assessment can distinguish invasive melanoma from coincident benign nevus, but immunohistochemistry may be required to differentiate desmoplastic melanoma from scar, remembering that S-100 cells are not uncommonly seen in dermal scars.[28,29]

Margin Assessment for Melanoma on Sun-Damaged Skin

Conventional (transverse, vertical) sections
Histologic assessment of peripheral margins of melanomas excised from sun-damaged skin usually involves examination for in situ melanoma (typically lentigo

Pitfalls
Lesions in specimen argins that mimic melanoma in situ

! Solar melanocytic hyperplasia

! Solar lentigines (eg, flat solar lentigo of facial skin)

! Field effect (melanocytic hyperplasia adjacent to melanoma)

! Melanocytic hyperplasia secondary to previous biopsy (overlying scar)

! Lichenoid reactions, especially those with pseudonest formation

maligna pattern). The horizontal, circumferential growth of LM is thought to occur by continuous, noninterrupted, subclinical spread of melanoma (in situ) cells at the dermal-epidermal junction.[7] Recurrence rates of 8% to 20% have been reported when conventional vertical transverse sections are used for margin assessment in head and neck melanoma,[30–33] and data in the literature suggest that routine use of a 5 mm margin for in situ melanoma on sun-damaged skin is inadequate.[34–36] Nevertheless, conventional radial sectioning at 1-mm intervals and second stage excision of positive margins, if required, has been successfully employed to achieve a 5% recurrence rate for LM and LMM (92% of cases on head and neck).[37]

En face sections

Because the horizontal spread of LM is continuous, en face margin assessment is considered by many to provide the best visualization of subclinical disease.[38] En face sections have been employed using many different techniques, including the use of oblique sections with MMS,[39] MMS followed by rush permanent sections,[36] slow MMS,[40] the square procedure,[41] and the Tübingen technique.[42]

Moehrle and colleagues[38] reported recurrence rates in 292 subjects who had lentigo maligna melanoma. Tumors recurred in 2.9% of 136 subjects whose lesion margins were assessed using en face formalin-fixed, paraffin-embedded sections. Only one of these subjects (0.7%) had a local recurrence. For 156 subjects treated using conventional histologic margin assessment, the recurrence rate was 17.9%, with 6.4% of subjects having a local recurrence.

The use of en face sections appears to give a lower recurrence rate and allows for narrower margins of excision. Disadvantages of en face sections include:

- Difficult to assess gradations of melanocytic hyperplasia
- Can be difficult to section and fully visualize margin if tissue fragments are curvilinear
- Not useful if lesion has a discontinuous growth pattern (eg, many cases of superficial spreading melanoma).[7]

Frozen sections

MMS employs en face frozen sections for margin assessment. En face frozen sections are also used in some institutions to assess margins during conventional surgical excision.[43] The use of frozen sections for margin assessment in lentigo maligna remains controversial. Several potential limitations have been identified:

- Artifacts in the frozen section (eg, folding)
- Difficulty differentiating keratinocytes and melanocytes
- Absence of significant retraction artifact around melanocytes
- Lack of reproducibility with multiple observers.[43]

Despite the lack of prospective, randomized, controlled studies on the utility of MMS for lentigo maligna and lentigo maligna melanoma, results published by experienced Mohs surgeons support the utility of frozen section in accurate margin assessment. For example, Zitelli and colleagues[39] have achieved a local recurrence rate of less than 0.5% using MMS and en face frozen sections. Examination of subsequent formalin-fixed, paraffin-embedded tissue shows good correlation with the frozen section slides.[35,44,45] Margins read as negative by the Mohs surgeon at frozen section were all confirmed as negative by a dermatopathologist on permanent section.[45] However, when difficult-to-interpret frozen sections are subsequently evaluated on permanent section, the sensitivity and specificity of frozen sections was only 59% and 81% respectively[46]; and the study by Prieto and colleagues[43] clearly shows that dermatopathologists have low concordance between frozen section and permanent section margin interpretation for melanocytic lesions.

USE OF IMMUNOHISTOCHEMISTRY FOR MARGIN ASSESSMENT

The use of immunohistochemical stains may allow for more accurate recognition of melanocytic proliferation in specimens from melanoma margins (**Fig. 5**).[47]

Melan-A/MART-1

The most commonly used antibody for assessment of melanoma margins is Melan-A (MART-1), which recognizes a premelanosomal antigen in cells of melanocyte lineage. Melan-A is sensitive and specific for melanocytes, but several pitfalls must be recognized. In intraepidermal melanocytic proliferations, Melan-A may stain adjacent

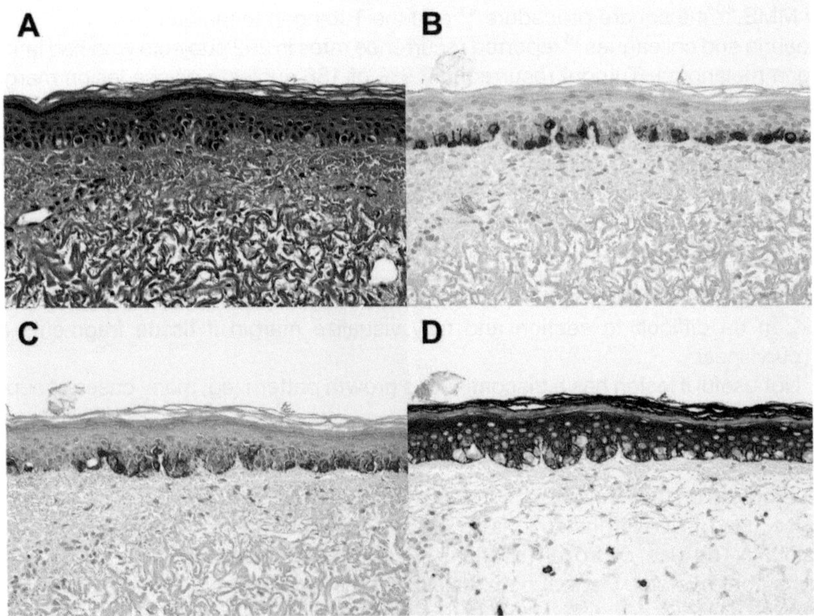

Fig. 5. Use of immunohistochemistry in the diagnosis of melanoma in situ. Foci of contiguous melanocytic hyperplasia are seen on the hematoxylin and eosin stain (*A*), and easily identified on Melan-A (*B*) and HMB45 (*C*) immunohistochemistry. Atypical melanocytes are also highlighted as large negative-staining cells using antikeratin antibodies (*D*).

keratinocytes, presumably secondary to antigen transfer, and Melan-A staining often overestimates the melanocyte density when compared, for example, with HMB45 staining.[27,48–50] Rarely, Melan-A positivity is found within the pseudonests of lichenoid reactions.[27] Finally, isolated Melan-A positive cells are sometimes found in the dermis of sun-damaged skin.[16] These cells do not appear to represent melanocytes and should not be over interpreted as invasive melanoma. A rapid method for Melan-A immunostaining may be employed on frozen sections used in Mohs micrographic surgery.[51]

Other Immunostains

S-100 is too nonspecific for use in assessment of intraepidermal melanocytic proliferations in this setting, especially because intraepidermal Langerhans cells are S-100 positive. HMB45, like Melan-A, is a specific melanocyte marker, but it is less sensitive. However, it may have less nonspecific keratinocyte staining than Melan-A. Microphthalmia transcription factor is a useful melanocyte marker and has the advantage that specific nuclear staining is more easily amenable to quantitative assessment of melanocytic hyperplasia, than is cytoplasmic staining with Melan-A, HMB45, or antibodies against tyrosinase.

SUMMARY

The more complete the pathologic examination of the surgical margins in a melanoma-excision specimen, the greater one's certainty that the lesion has been completely excised. Bread-loaf or en face methods, or a combination, can be used to assess melanoma margins. En face sectioning, despite some shortcomings, allows assessment of close to 100% of the peripheral margins without requiring examination of hundreds of tissues sections.

In sun-damaged skin, the evaluation of melanoma margins is particularly problematic because of co-incident lesions that mimic melanoma and background melanocytic hyperplasia caused by prolonged sun-exposure (solar melanocytic hyperplasia). When strict criteria are employed (contiguous melanocytic hyperplasia, nesting, or pagetoid spread), melanoma in situ can be reliably detected within the margins of an excision specimen, in formalin-fixed, paraffin-embedded tissue, and in frozen sections, used, for example, in Mohs micrographic surgery. Although the detection of atypical melanocytic hyperplasia is problematic on frozen sections, clinical follow-up data suggest that this pattern of melanocytic hyperplasia, even if present in a surgical margin, may not be biologically significant in lesion recurrence.

Finally, immunohistochemistry, especially using the Melan-A (MART-1) antibody may be a useful ancillary technique allowing identification of melanoma in situ in tissue sections.

REFERENCES

1. Cochran AJ. Prudent margins for melanocytic lesions. Eur J Plast Surg 2001;24: 78–9.
2. Abide JM, Nahai F, Bennet RG. The meaning of surgical margins. Plast Reconstr Surg 1984;73:492–6.
3. Bennett RG. The meaning and significance of tissue margins. Adv Dermatol 1989;4:343–55.
4. Rapini RP. Comparison of methods for checking surgical margins. J Am Acad Dermatol 1990;23:288–94.

5. Shriner DL, McCoy DK, Goldberg DJ, et al. Mohs micrographic surgery. J Am Acad Dermatol 1998;39:79–97.
6. Kimyai-Asadi A, Katz T, Goldberg LH, et al. Margin involvement after the excision of melanoma in situ: the need for complete en face examination of the surgical margins. Dermatol Surg 2007;33:1434–9.
7. Breuninger H, Schlagenhauff B, Stroebel W, et al. Patterns of local horizontal spread of melanomas: consequences for surgery and histopathologic evaluation. Am J Surg Pathol 1999;23:1493–8.
8. Barnhill RL, Piepkorn M, Busam KJ. Pathology of melanocytic nevi and malignant melanoma. 2nd edition. New York: Springer; 2004. p. 278.
9. Agarwal-Antal N, Bowen GM, Gerwels JW. Histologic evaluation of lentigo maligna with permanent sections: implications regarding current guidelines. J Am Acad Dermatol 2002;47:743–8.
10. Ackerman AB, Briggs PL, Bravo F. Differential diagnosis in dermatopathology III. Philadelphia: Lea & Febiger; 1993. p. 166–9.
11. Weyers W, Bonczkowitz M, Weyers I, et al. Melanoma in situ versus melanocytic hyperplasia in sun-damaged skin: assessment of the significance of histopathologic criteria for the differential diagnosis. Am J Dermatopathol 1996;18:560–6.
12. Acker SM, Nicholson JH, Rust PF, et al. Morphometric discrimination of melanoma in situ of sun-damaged skin from chronically sun-damaged skin. J Am Acad Dermatol 1998;39:239–45.
13. Barlow JO, Maize JM Sr, Lang PG. The density and distribution of melanocytes adjacent to melanoma and non-melanoma skin cancers. Dermatol Surg 2007;33:199–207.
14. Cohen LM. The starburst giant cell is useful for distinguishing lentigo maligna from photodamaged skin. J Am Acad Dermatol 1996;35:962–8.
15. Farrahi F, Egbert BM, Swetter SM. Histologic similarities between lentigo maligna and dysplastic nevus: importance of clinicopathologic distinction. J Cutan Pathol 2005;32:405–12.
16. Hendi A, Brodland DG, Zitelli JA. Melanocytes in long-standing sun-exposed skin. Quantitative analysis using the MART-1 immunostain. Arch Dermatol 2006;142:871–6.
17. Andersen WK, Labadie RR, Bhawan J. Histopathology of solar lentigines of the face: a quantitative study. J Am Acad Dermatol 1997;36:444–7.
18. Dalton SR, Gardner TL, Libow LF, et al. Contiguous lesions in lentigo maligna. J Am Acad Dermatol 2005;52:859–62.
19. Somach SC, Taira JW, Pitha JV, et al. Pigmented lesions in actinically damaged skin. Histopathologic comparison of biopsy and excisional specimens. Arch Dermatol 1996;132:1297–302.
20. Wong CK. A study of melanocytes in the normal skin surrounding malignant melanoma. Dermatologica 1970;141:215–25.
21. Fallowfield ME, Cook MG. Epidermal melanocytes adjacent to melanoma and the field change effect. Histopathology 1990;17:397–400.
22. Bastian BC, Kashani-Sabet M, Hamm H, et al. Gene amplifications characterize acral melanoma and permit the detection of occult tumor cells in the surrounding skin. Cancer Res 2000;60:1968–73.
23. North JP, Kageshita T, Pinkel D, et al. Distribution and significance of occult intraepidermal tumor cells surrounding primary melanoma. J Invest Dermatol 2008;128:2024–30.
24. Fallowfield ME, Cook MG. Re-excisions of scar in primary cutaneous melanoma: a histopathological study. Br J Dermatol 1992;126:47–51.

25. Duve S, Schmoeckel C, Burgdorf W. Melanocytic hyperplasia in scars: a histopathological investigation of 722 cases. Am J Dermatopathol 1996;18:236–40.
26. Dalton SR, Baptista MA, Libow LF, et al. Lichenoid tissue reaction in malignant melanoma, a potential diagnostic pitfall. Am J Clin Pathol 2002;117:766–70.
27. Maize JC, Resneck JS, Shapiro PE, et al. Ducking stray "magic bullets": a Melan-A alert. Am J Dermatopathol 2003;25:162–5.
28. Robson A, Allen P, Hollowood K. S100 expression in cutaneous scars: a potential diagnostic pitfall in the diagnosis of desmoplastic melanoma. Histopathology 2001;38:135–40.
29. Chorny JA, Barr RJ. S100-positive spindle cells in scars: a diagnostic pitfall in the re-excision of desmoplastic melanoma. Am J Dermatopathol 2002;24:309–12.
30. Pitman GH, Kopf AW, Bart RS, et al. Treatment of lentigo maligna and lentigo maligna melanoma. J Dermatol Surg Oncol 1979;5:727–37.
31. Coleman WP III, Davis RS, Reed RJ, et al. Treatment of lentigo maligna and lentigo maligna melanoma. J Dermatol Surg Oncol 1980;6:476–9.
32. Karakousis CP, Balch CM, Urist MM, et al. Local recurrence in malignant melanoma: long term results of the multiinstitutional randomized surgical trial. Ann Surg Oncol 1996;3:446–52.
33. Osborne JE, Hutchinson PE. A follow-up study to investigate the efficacy of initial treatment of lentigo maligna with surgical excision. Br J Plast Surg 2002;55:611–5.
34. Zitelli JA, Brown CD, Hanusa BH. Surgical margins for excision of primary cutaneous melanoma. J Am Acad Dermatol 1997;37:422–9.
35. Robinson JK. Margin control for lentigo maligna. J Am Acad Dermatol 1994;31: 79–85.
36. Cohen LM, McCall MW, Hodge SJ, et al. Successful treatment of lentigo maligna and lentigo maligna melanoma with Mohs micrographic surgery aided by rush permanent sections. Cancer 1994;73:2964–70.
37. Bub JL, Berg D, Slee A, et al. Management of lentigo maligna and lentigo maligna melanoma with staged excision. A 5-year follow-up. Arch Dermatol 2004;140: 552–8.
38. Moehrle M, Dietz K, Garbe C, et al. Conventional histology vs. three-dimensional histology in lentigo maligna melanoma. Br J Dermatol 2006;154:453–9.
39. Zitelli JA, Brown CD, Hanusa BH. Mohs micrographic surgery for the treatment of primary cutaneous melanoma. J Am Acad Dermatol 1997;37:236–45.
40. Clayton BD, Leshin B, Hitchcock MG, et al. Utility of rush paraffin-embedded tangential sections in the management of cutaneous neoplasms. Dermatol Surg 2000;26:671–8.
41. Johnson TM, Headington JT, Baker SR, et al. Usefulness of the staged excision for lentigo maligna and lentigo maligna melanoma: the "square procedure". J Am Acad Dermatol 1997;37:758–64.
42. Breuninger H, Schaumberg-Lever G. Control of excisional margins by conventional histopathological techniques in the treatment of skin tumours. An alternative to the Mohs' technique. J Pathol 1988;154:167–71.
43. Prieto VG, Argenyi ZB, Barnhill RB, et al. Are en face frozen sections accurate for diagnosing margin status in melanocytic lesions? Am J Clin Pathol 2003;120: 203–8.
44. Zitelli JA, Moy RL, Abell E. The reliability of frozen sections in the evaluation of surgical margins for melanoma. J Am Acad Dermatol 1991;24:102–6.
45. Bienert TN, Trotter MJ, Arlette JP. Treatment of cutaneous melanoma of the face by Mohs micrographic surgery. J Cutan Med Surg 2003;7:25–30.

46. Barlow RJ, White CR, Swanson NA. Mohs' micrographic surgery using frozen sections alone may be unsuitable for detecting single atypical melanocytes at the margins of melanoma in situ. Br J Dermatol 2002;146:290–4.
47. Thosani MK, Marghoob A, Chen CSJ. Current progress in immunostains in Mohs micrographic surgery: a review. Dermatol Surg 2008;34:1621–36.
48. El Shabrawi-Caelen L, Kerl H, Cerroni L. Melan-A: not a helpful marker in distinction between melanoma in situ on sun-damaged skin and pigmented actinic keratosis. Am J Dermatopathol 2004;26:364–6.
49. Wlitz KL, Qureshi H, Patterson JW, et al. Immunostaining for MART-1 in interpretation of problematic intra-epidermal pigmented lesions. J Cutan Pathol 2007;34: 601–5.
50. Helm K, Findeis-Hosey J. Immunohistochemistry of pigmented actinic keratoses, actinic keratoses, melanoma in situ and solar lentigines with Melan-A. J Cutan Pathol 2008;35:931–4.
51. Kelley LC, Starkus L. Immunohistochemical staining of lentigo maligna during Mohs micrographic surgery using MART-1. J Am Acad Dermatol 2002;46:78–84.

Sentinel Lymph Nodes in Cutaneous Melanoma

Victor G. Prieto, MD, PhD

KEYWORDS

• Melanoma • Sentinel lymph node • Immunoperoxidase
• Capsular nevus • Tumor burden

SENTINEL LYMPH NODES

Overview

Although not all authors consider sentinel lymph nodes (SLN) to be standard of care in patients who have cutaneous melanoma, it is true that within the last 10 years evaluation of SLN has probably become the most popular method of early staging of patients who are oncologic. Because SLN are considered to be the lymph nodes most likely to contain metastatic deposits, the pathologist can examine them in a more intense manner than in standard lymphadenectomy specimens (single, routine hematoxylin, and eosin section per paraffin block). Although it has been suggested that removal of SLN may improve overall survival, currently the main goal of examination of SLN is to provide staging information, by more accurately defining the prognosis of these patients and providing more consistent grouping in clinical trials. This issue will discuss the main clinical, gross, histologic, and immunohistochemical features of SLN examination in patients who have cutaneous melanoma.

Gross Features

Before discussing the processing of SLN, the clinical criteria used to recommend SLN examination has to be discussed. Most protocols recommend SLN examination in patients who have melanomas with Breslow thickness 1 mm or greater or with ulceration. In addition, many protocols also include Clark level IV. At the author's institution, lesions with vertical growth phase (in particular those cases with dermal mitotic figures), vascular invasion, and satellitosis are also considered as criteria for SLN examination. It is unclear if the presence of regression correlates with a higher rate of positive SLN,[1] so most protocols do not consider regression as an criterion for SLN analysis.

A version of this article was previously published in *Surgical Pathology Clinics* 2:3.
Departments of Pathology and Dermatology, University of Texas, MD Anderson Cancer Center, 1515 Holcombe Boulevard Unit 85, Houston, TX 77030, USA
E-mail address: vprieto@mdanderson.org

Clin Lab Med 31 (2011) 301–310
doi:10.1016/j.cll.2011.03.007
labmed.theclinics.com
0272-2712/11/$ – see front matter

Key Features
Reporting

Possible prognostic factors of metastasis to sentinel lymph nodes

1. Larger size (in millimeter)
2. Intraparenchymal location
3. Extracapsular extension

Frozen sections have been used in SLN to try to render an immediate diagnosis of metastatic melanoma during the surgical procedure. Those patients who have positive SLN by frozen section would then undergo completion of the regional lymph nodes in the same surgical procedure; however, frozen sections provide a suboptimal morphology and may not contain the subcapsular region of the lymph node (likely area of early involvement by melanoma). Furthermore, since processing of the frozen tissue requires embedding and new sectioning of the paraffin block, it is possible that small, micrometastases are lost in the unexamined tissue.[2] Therefore, at least for SLN from patients who have melanoma, most authors consider examination of routinely processed material (formalin-fixed, paraffin-embedded) as gold standard and do not recommend frozen sections. An alternative is touch preparations/cytologic specimens,[3,4] however, it is not a widespread technique probably because of the sometimes difficult distinction between melanoma cells and pigmented macrophages.

Regarding grossing techniques, there is no complete agreement in how to process SLN. However, it has become apparent that the classical processing used for nonsentinel lymph nodes (ie, bivalving of the node and examination of a single, routine hematoxylin and eosin [H&E] slide), is not sensitive enough. In an early study from the author's institution with 243 subjects who had SLN initially diagnosed negative when examining one H&E slide per block, 10 subjects (4.3%) presented a recurrence in the same lymphatic basin. Of those 10 subjects, when the original SLN was reexamined using new serial sections or immunohistochemistry, eight (80%) were reclassified as positive.[5] In another study, three of seven subjects with recurrent disease had metastatic melanoma in the originally negative SLN after reexamination with serial sections and immunohistochemistry.[6] Based upon these studies, most current protocols for examination of SLN require more than one hematoxylin and eosin section or addition of immunohistochemistry.

The original protocol proposed by Cochran[7] called for bivalving the SLN through the hilum with the intent to allow examination of the lymphatic vessels of the lymph node. At the author's institution, breadloafing of the SLN is recommended to allow examination of a large area of the subcapsular region (**Fig. 1**),[8] then one H&E slide is studied, if this is positive it is reported as such or else the block is submitted to the laboratory again to obtain a new H&E deeper section slide (~200 microns deeper in the block) and two unstained slides. One of them is reacted with a panmelanocytic cocktail (HMB45, anti-MART1, and antityrosinase) and the other is left in case additional studies are needed.

An alternative processing of SLN, in the context of some clinical trials, calls for preserving a portion of the node for polymerase chain reaction (PCR) analysis.

CUTANEOUS MELANOMA IN SENTINEL LYMPH NODES

Microscopic Features

Approximately 20% of patients who have cutaneous melanoma show deposits of melanoma cells in the SLN. The amount of tumor in the SLN (tumor burden) ranges

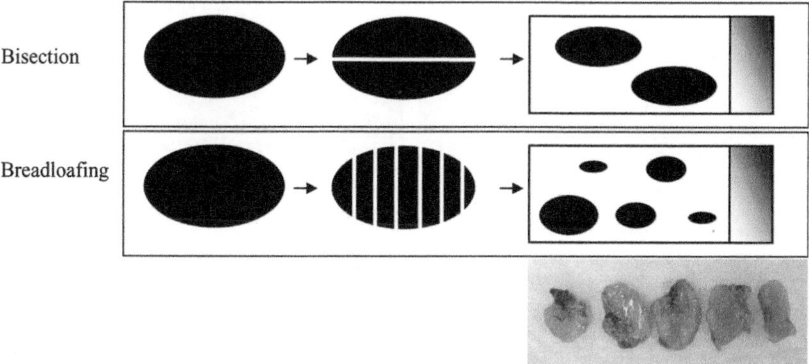

Fig. 1. Main techniques used to gross sentinel lymph nodes. At MDACC the protocols call for breadloafing and include as many fragments as possible within a single paraffin block.

from solitary, rare cells to complete replacement of the lymph node. The majority of metastatic melanoma deposits are located within, or close to, the subcapsular sinus (**Fig. 2**). Less frequently, tumor cells are located within the parenchyma closer to the center of the lymph node (**Fig. 3**) and even rarely (<5% of cases) there is extracapsular extension into the perinodal fibroadipose tissues.

Metastatic melanoma cells may display a large variety of morphologies, although most commonly they resemble the cells in the primary lesion. At the time of examination of SLN, it is very important to study the original melanoma, particularly to distinguish metastatic cells from macrophages or nevus cells.

Immunohistochemical studies are helpful when trying to detect small metastatic deposits and also at the time of differential diagnosis. Of the approximately 20% of patients who have metastasis to the SLN, 16% are detected in the initial hematoxylin and eosin slide and the remaining 4% are detected with the serial sections or immunoperoxidase. Some authors propose the use of anti-S100 protein.[9,10] However, in addition to melanoma cells, this marker also labels nevus cells and lymph node dendritic cells. The resulting high background staining limits the practical utility of this immunohistochemical stain in this setting. Therefore most authors recommend the use of other markers.[11,12] Among the different options, the author agrees with the recommendation of using a pan-melanocytic cocktail (HMB45, anti-MART1, and

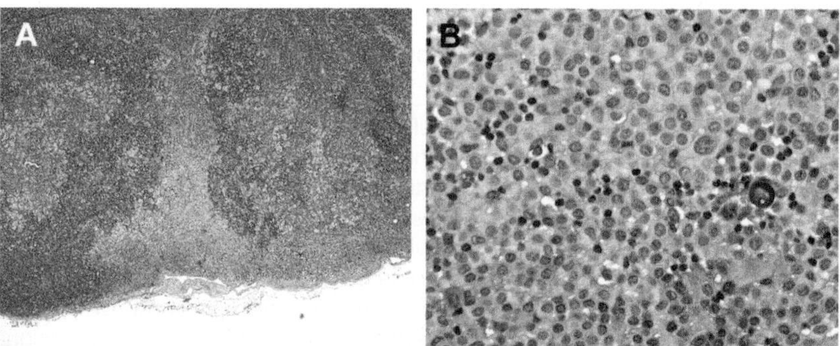

Fig. 2. (*A*) Cluster of metastatic melanoma involving the subcapsular region. (*B*) Note the large size, irregular nuclear contour, and prominent nucleoli.

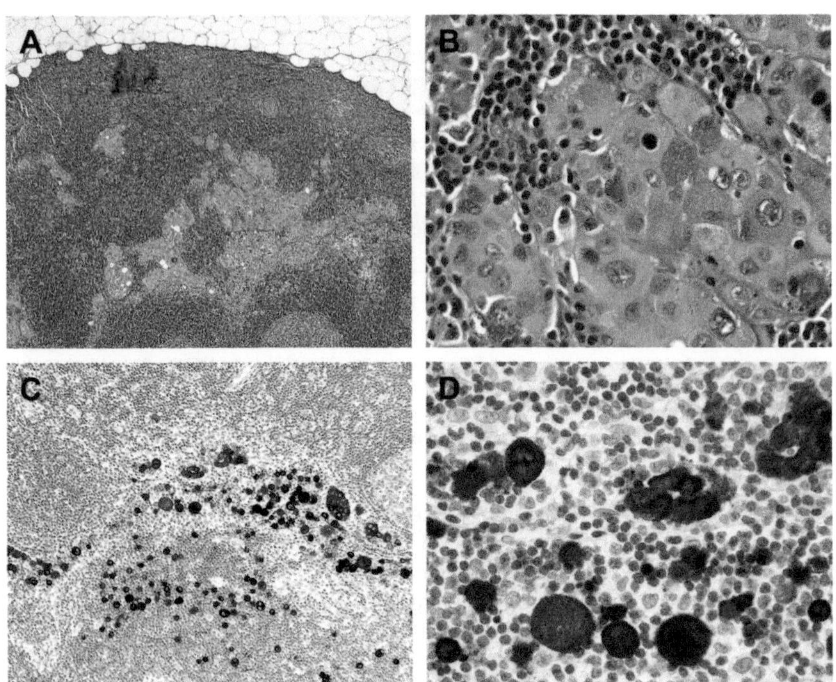

Fig. 3. (*A*) Metastatic melanoma to intraparenchymal location. (*B*) Higher magnification reveals the large nuclei and prominent nucleoli. (*C*) Melanoma cells react with a panmelanocytic cocktail (panmelanocytic cocktail: HMB45, anti-MART1, and anti-tyrosinase; diaminobencidine and light hematoxylin). (*D*) Melanoma cells as described in 3(*C*) at high magnification.

antityrosinase [see **Fig. 3**]) to increase the detection of tumor cells.[13] Occasionally the author uses HMB45 by itself when trying to differentiate between macrophages and melanoma cells (see differential diagnosis discussion). The only situation in which the author uses anti-S100 is for those cases of melanoma (usually spindle cell type) in which the tumor cells do not express MART1 or gp100 (with HMB45). Furthermore, the lack of expression of MART1 in a spindle cell melanocytic proliferation supports a diagnosis of melanoma.[14]

MELANOMA CELLS IN SENTINEL LYMPH NODES

Differential Diagnosis

In general, it is easy to detect melanoma cells in SLN. Such cells are usually large, with prominent nucleoli, focal cytoplasmic melanin pigment, and are arranged in clusters in the subcapsular region. However, and particularly in those cases in which there are isolated tumor cells, it may be difficult to distinguish them from macrophages or large lymphocytes. As mentioned, comparison with the original cutaneous melanoma may be helpful when trying to distinguish melanoma cells from macrophages. Also, immunohistochemical studies are helpful because the immense majority of metastatic melanoma cells to SLN will label for melanocytic markers. However, occasionally macrophages will label with anti-MART1[15]; therefore, if there are any doubts of isolated cells labeled with anti-MART1 actually being macrophages and not melanoma cells, the author recommends using HMB45 by itself (in the author's experience macrophages labeled with HMB45 are rarely seen).[14]

The differential diagnosis also includes capsular nevi. These are clusters of benign melanocytes, most commonly present in the lymph node capsule. Up to 20% of lymphadenectomies from the axilla or groin contain such melanocytes.[16] The capsular location of these nevus deposits is different from the subcapsular location of metastatic melanoma (**Fig. 4**). However, a potential problem is the presence of vascular metastasis detected in the intracapsular lymphatic vessels of the node. In such cases, use of anti-CD31, anti-CD34, or D2-40 may be helpful in detecting the rim of endothelial cells around the melanoma clusters, thus confirming the intravascular location. On the other hand, rarely capsular nevi extend into the underlying node parenchyma. In general, those lymph nodes contain similar melanocytes in the capsular region, lack gp100 expression (with HMB45), and show very low Ki67 expression.[17,18]

Diagnosis

As mentioned, if the original hematoxylin and eosin slide is negative, the author examines a deeper hematoxylin and eosin slide and an immunoperoxidase slide labeled with the panmelanocytic cocktail. Then the author issues a diagnosis including the number of positive nodes and the total count (see diagnostic algorithm, **Fig. 5**). To avoid possible typographical errors, the author recommends using the numbers and spelling (eg, one of two lymph nodes [1/2]). In addition, quantification of the amount of melanoma deposits in the SLN appears to provide prognostic information (see later discussion). Based upon the author's results,[19] the author now measures the amount

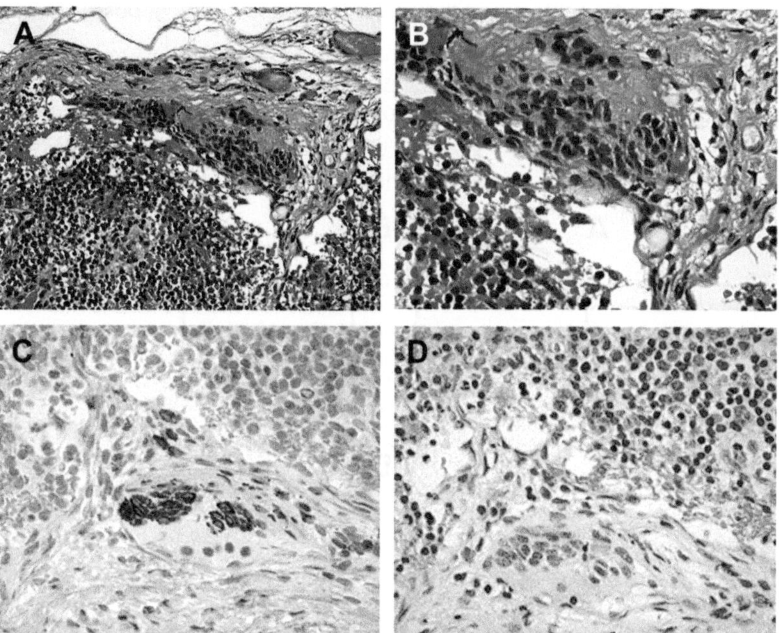

Fig. 4. (*A*) Nodal nevus. Notice the small melanocytes located in the capsule of the SLN. (*B*) At higher power these cells show uniform nuclei with small nucleoli. Mitotic figures are not evident. These cells express MART1. (*C*) but not gp100 (*D*) ([*C*]: anti-MART1 with light hematoxylin; [*D*]: HMB45 with light hematoxylin).

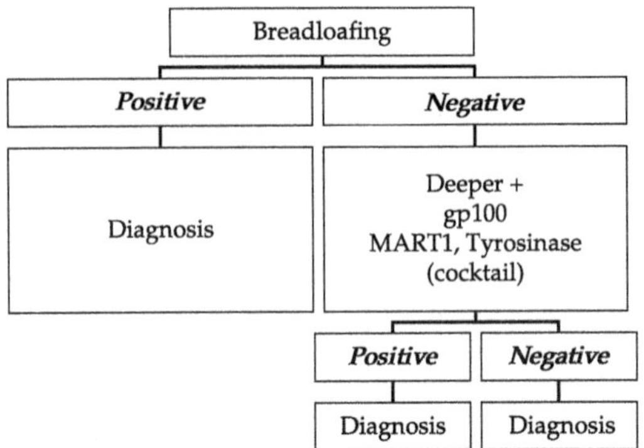

Fig. 5. Diagnostic algorithm used at MDACC. If the initial hematoxylin and eosin is negative, the block is recut (after approximately 200 μm) in three sections. One is stained with hematoxylin and eosin and another with a panmelanocytic cocktail against gp100 (with HMB45), MART1, and tyrosinase.

of melanoma cells seen in the SLN as the size of the largest tumor deposit (in two dimensions, in millimeter), the location (subcapsular versus intraparenchymal/mixed subcapsular/intraparenchymal), and presence or absence of extracapsular extension (**Fig. 6**, also see later discussion on prognosis). For the purpose of measuring, when small aggregates are located in clusters in the same region of the SLN, the author considers them to be a single nest. This practice of quantifying the amount of metastatic melanoma seems to be extending because a recent survey in Europe has shown that a majority of participants report the size of the largest tumor deposit in the SLN.[20]

Prognosis

Multiple studies have confirmed that SLN positivity is associated with impaired prognosis, along with Breslow thickness, and ulceration.[21–24] Recent studies have shown

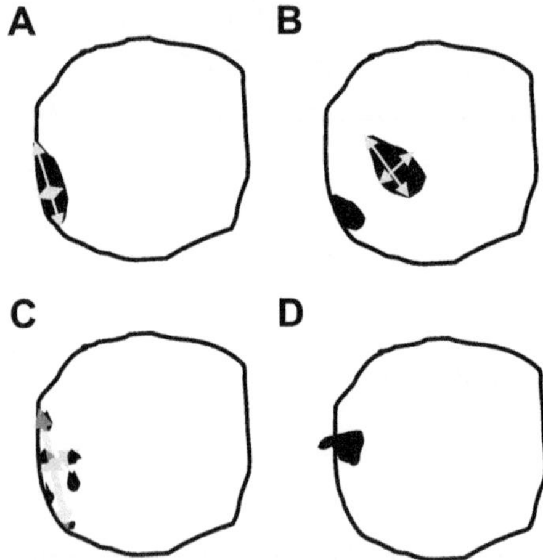

Fig. 6. (*A*) Measurement of a subcapsular nest. (*B*) Subcapsular and intraparenchymal nests. The larger is measured. (*C*) Cluster of small nests measured in aggregate. (*D*) Presence of extracapsular extension.

Pitfalls
Sentinel lymph nodes

! Macrophages can be labeled with anti-MART1.

! Capsular nevi can also (rarely) involve the node parenchyma.

! Spindle cell melanoma can be negative for gp100 (with HMB45) and MART1. Use an additional anti-S100 in such cases.

that quantification of the amount of melanoma in SLN correlates with subsequent involvement of nonsentinel lymph nodes, from the completion lymphadenectomy specimens,[25–31] and furthermore, with prognosis.[19,27,32–36] The two main techniques suggested to perform this quantification are a modification of Breslow thickness (measurement of the distance between the capsule and the most deeply located deposit) and measurement of the size of the tumor deposits (in millimeter, in one or two dimensions).

The author's preliminary data on 237 positive SLN out of 1417 patients,[19] suggest a stratification in three groups with progressively worse prognosis:

1. Involvement of one or two SLN and metastasis size 2mm or smaller (in the largest nest), and no ulceration (in the primary lesion)
2. Ulceration in the primary lesion or metastasis size greater than 2 mm (in the largest nest)
3. Involvement of three or more SLN or ulceration in the primary lesion and metastasis size greater than 2 mm (in the largest nest).

An important finding in the author's study was the lack of a cutoff in the metastasis size associated with no risk of subsequent metastasis. The author has seen at least two cases in which only a single melanoma cell was identified in the SLN that recurred with multiple distant metastases within 4 years of diagnosis.

Some studies have indicated that detection of melanocytic mRNA in SLN by PCR correlates with decreased survival,[37–39] but other authors have not found significant differences.[40,41] A possible explanation for these differences may be the presence of nodal nevi in some SLN. Thus, even though it seems logical that detection of melanocytic mRNA in SLN should correlate with worse prognosis, it is likely that at least some of the SLN with positive PCR actually correspond to capsular nevi and not to metastatic melanoma deposits. Therefore, unless mRNA specific for melanoma cells becomes available for PCR studies, it seems that histologic examination will remain the gold standard in SLN for melanoma.

In summary, SLN is becoming a widespread technique to stage patients who have cutaneous melanoma. Ongoing studies are addressing the possible therapeutic effect secondary to the removal of positive SLN.

REFERENCES

1. Kaur C, Thomas RJ, Desai N, et al. The correlation of regression in primary melanoma with sentinel lymph node status. J Clin Pathol 2008;61(3):297–300.
2. Prieto VG. Use of frozen sections in the examination of sentinel lymph nodes in patients with melanoma. Semin Diagn Pathol 2008;25(2):112–5.
3. Messina JL, Glass LF, Cruse CW, et al. Pathologic examination of the sentinel lymph node in malignant melanoma. Am J Surg Pathol 1999;23(6):686–90.

4. Creager AJ, Shiver SA, Shen P, et al. Intraoperative evaluation of sentinel lymph nodes for metastatic melanoma by imprint cytology. Cancer 2002;94(11):3016–22.
5. Gershenwald JE, Colome MI, Lee JE, et al. Patterns of recurrence following a negative sentinel lymph node biopsy in 243 patients with stage I or II melanoma. J Clin Oncol 1998;16(6):2253–60.
6. Clary BM, Brady MS, Lewis JJ, et al. Sentinel lymph node biopsy in the management of patients with primary cutaneous melanoma: review of a large single-institutional experience with an emphasis on recurrence. Ann Surg 2001;233(2):250–8.
7. Cochran AJ. Surgical pathology remains pivotal in the evaluation of 'sentinel' lymph nodes. Am J Surg Pathol 1999;23(10):1169–72.
8. Prieto VG, Clark SH. Processing of sentinel lymph nodes for detection of metastatic melanoma. Ann Diagn Pathol 2002;6(4):257–64.
9. Gibbs JF, Huang PP, Zhang PJ, et al. Accuracy of pathologic techniques for the diagnosis of metastatic melanoma in sentinel lymph nodes. Ann Surg Oncol 1999;6(7):699–704.
10. Yu LL, Flotte TJ, Tanabe KK, et al. Detection of microscopic melanoma metastases in sentinel lymph nodes. Cancer 1999;86(4):617–27.
11. Shidham VB, Qi DY, Acker S, et al. Evaluation of micrometastases in sentinel lymph nodes of cutaneous melanoma: higher diagnostic accuracy with Melan-A and MART-1 compared with S-100 protein and HMB-45. Am J Surg Pathol 2001;25(8):1039–46.
12. Abrahamsen HN, Hamilton-Dutoit SJ, Larsen J, et al. Sentinel lymph nodes in malignant melanoma: extended histopathologic evaluation improves diagnostic precision. Cancer 2004;100(8):1683–91.
13. Shidham VB, Qi D, Rao RN, et al. Improved immunohistochemical evaluation of micrometastases in sentinel lymph nodes of cutaneous melanoma with 'MCW Melanoma Cocktail' - a mixture of monoclonal antibodies to MART-1, melan-A, and tyrosinase. BMC Cancer 2003;3(1):15.
14. Prieto VG, Shea CR. Use of immunohistochemistry in melanocytic lesions. J Cutan Pathol 2008;35(Suppl 2):1–10.
15. Trejo O, Reed JA, Prieto VG. Atypical cells in human cutaneous re-excision scars for melanoma express p75NGFR, C56/N-CAM and GAP-43: evidence of early Schwann cell differentiation. J Cutan Pathol 2002;29(7):397–406.
16. Carson KF, Wen DR, Li PX, et al. Nodal nevi and cutaneous melanomas. Am J Surg Pathol 1996;20(7):834–40.
17. Lohmann CM, Iversen K, Jungbluth AA, et al. Expression of melanocyte differentiation antigens and ki-67 in nodal nevi and comparison of ki-67 expression with metastatic melanoma. Am J Surg Pathol 2002;26(10):1351–7.
18. Biddle DA, Evans HL, Kemp BL, et al. Intraparenchymal nevus cell aggregates in lymph nodes: a possible diagnostic pitfall with malignant melanoma and carcinoma. Am J Surg Pathol 2003;27(5):673–81.
19. Prieto VG, Diwan AD, Lazar AFJ, et al. Histologic quantification of tumor size in sentinel lymph node metastases correlates with prognosis in patients with cutaneous malignant melanoma. Mod Pathol 2006;19(Suppl1):87A.
20. Batistatou A, Cook MG, Massi D. Histopathology report of cutaneous melanoma and sentinel lymph node in Europe: a web-based survey by the dermatopathology Working Group of the European Society of Pathology. Virchows Arch 2009; 454(5):505–11.
21. Cascinelli N, Belli F, Santinami M, et al. Sentinel lymph node biopsy in cutaneous melanoma: the WHO Melanoma Program experience. Ann Surg Oncol 2000;7(6): 469–74.

22. Gershenwald JE, Thompson W, Mansfield PF, et al. Multi-institutional melanoma lymphatic mapping experience: the prognostic value of sentinel lymph node status in 612 stage I or II melanoma patients. J Clin Oncol 1999;17(3):976–83.
23. Rousseau DL Jr, Ross MI, Johnson MM, et al. Revised American Joint Committee on Cancer staging criteria accurately predict sentinel lymph node positivity in clinically node-negative melanoma patients. Ann Surg Oncol 2003;10(5):569–74.
24. Topping A, Dewar D, Rose V, et al. Five years of sentinel node biopsy for melanoma: the St George's Melanoma Unit experience. Br J Plast Surg 2004;57(2): 97–104.
25. Frankel TL, Griffith KA, Lowe L, et al. Do micromorphometric features of metastatic deposits within sentinel nodes predict nonsentinel lymph node involvement in melanoma? Ann Surg Oncol 2008;15(9):2403–11.
26. Page AJ, Carlson GW, Delman KA, et al. Prediction of nonsentinel lymph node involvement in patients with a positive sentinel lymph node in malignant melanoma. Am Surg 2007;73(7):674–8 [discussion: 678–9].
27. Debarbieux S, Duru G, Dalle S, et al. Sentinel lymph node biopsy in melanoma: a micromorphometric study relating to prognosis and completion lymph node dissection. Br J Dermatol 2007;157(1):58–67.
28. Sabel MS, Griffith K, Sondak VK, et al. Predictors of nonsentinel lymph node positivity in patients with a positive sentinel node for melanoma. J Am Coll Surg 2005; 201(1):37–47.
29. Gershenwald JE, Andtbacka RH, Prieto VG, et al. Microscopic tumor burden in sentinel lymph nodes predicts synchronous nonsentinel lymph node involvement in patients with melanoma. J Clin Oncol 2008;26(26):4296–303.
30. Guggenheim M, Dummer R, Jung FJ, et al. The influence of sentinel lymph node tumour burden on additional lymph node involvement and disease-free survival in cutaneous melanoma–a retrospective analysis of 392 cases. Br J Cancer 2008; 98(12):1922–8.
31. Dewar DJ, Newell B, Green MA, et al. The microanatomic location of metastatic melanoma in sentinel lymph nodes predicts nonsentinel lymph node involvement. J Clin Oncol 2004;22(16):3345–9.
32. Rossi CR, De Salvo GL, Bonandini E, et al. Factors predictive of nonsentinel lymph node involvement and clinical outcome in melanoma patients with metastatic sentinel lymph node. Ann Surg Oncol 2008;15(4):1202–10.
33. van Akkooi AC, Bouwhuis MG, de Wilt JH, et al. Multivariable analysis comparing outcome after sentinel node biopsy or therapeutic lymph node dissection in patients with melanoma. Br J Surg 2007;94(10):1293–9.
34. Wright BE, Scheri RP, Ye X, et al. Importance of sentinel lymph node biopsy in patients with thin melanoma. Arch Surg 2008;143(9):892–9 [discussion: 899–900].
35. Guggenheim MM, Hug U, Jung FJ, et al. Morbidity and recurrence after completion lymph node dissection following sentinel lymph node biopsy in cutaneous malignant melanoma. Ann Surg 2008;247(4):687–93.
36. Satzger I, Völker B, Al Ghazal M, et al. Prognostic significance of histopathological parameters in sentinel nodes of melanoma patients. Histopathology 2007; 50(6):764–72.
37. Romanini A, Manca G, Pellegrino D, et al. Molecular staging of the sentinel lymph node in melanoma patients: correlation with clinical outcome. Ann Oncol 2005; 16(11):1832–40.
38. Gradilone A, Ribuffo D, Silvestri I, et al. Detection of melanoma cells in sentinel lymph nodes by reverse transcriptase-polymerase chain reaction: prognostic significance. Ann Surg Oncol 2004;11(11):983–7.

39. Mocellin S, Hoon DS, Pilati P, et al. Sentinel lymph node molecular ultrastaging in patients with melanoma: a systematic review and meta-analysis of prognosis. J Clin Oncol 2007;25(12):1588–95.
40. Scoggins CR, Ross MI, Reintgen DS, et al. Prospective multi-institutional study of reverse transcriptase polymerase chain reaction for molecular staging of melanoma. J Clin Oncol 2006;24(18):2849–57.
41. Hershko DD, Robb BW, Lowy AM, et al. Sentinel lymph node biopsy in thin melanoma patients. J Surg Oncol 2006;93(4):279–85.

Spitz Nevi, Atypical Spitzoid Neoplasms, and Spitzoid Melanoma

Daniel C. Zedek, MD, Timothy H. McCalmont, MD*

KEYWORDS

• Spitz nevus • Melanoma • Atypical spitzoid tumor
• Melanoma of childhood • FISH • Genomic

OVERVIEW

The distinction of Spitz nevi from melanoma remains one of the most challenging determinations facing the dermatopathologist today. Spitz nevi are benign neoplasms composed of large spindled or epithelioid melanocytes that commonly develop in the first two decades of life.[1] They can occur in any ethnic group and at any topographic location, but show a predilection for the faces of young children and thighs of young women with fair skin.

Spitzoid melanomas represent malignant melanocytic lesions with architectural and cytologic attributes overlapping those of Spitz nevi.[2] The determination as to what spitzoid is and what it is not can be subjective. Most spitzoid melanomas develop in adulthood, but occurrence in childhood and adolescence is also well documented. Spitzoid melanomas are not known to have any site predilection.

Atypical spitzoid neoplasms (also known as atypical Spitz tumors or atypical Spitz nevi) represent a controversial and incompletely defined diagnostic categorization. The designation is used by some to describe lesions with architecture and cytomorphology that is intermediate between Spitz nevi and spitzoid melanoma.[3] Typically these are lesions exhibiting many attributes of Spitz nevi but also displaying architectural atypicality, such as a lack of circumscription or defects in maturation, or cytologic atypicality, such as marked nucleomegaly, nuclear pleomorphism, or cells captured in mitosis. Many lesions within this spectrum are diagnostically controversial when shared amongst various experts and lack sufficient atypicality for a confident or unequivocal diagnosis of spitzoid melanoma, particularly in young patients. The

A version of this article was previously published in *Surgical Pathology Clinics* 2:3.
There are no funding sources and no conflicts of interest to disclose.
University of California, San Francisco, Dermatopathology, 1701 Divisadero Street, Suite 350, San Francisco, CA 94115, USA
* Corresponding author.
E-mail address: tim.mccalmont@ucsf.edu

Clin Lab Med 31 (2011) 311–320
doi:10.1016/j.cll.2011.03.008

Key Features
Spitz nevi, Spitzoid melanomas, Spitzoid neoplasms

1. Spitz nevi are benign proliferations of enlarged melanocytes with spindled or epithelioid cytomorphology that can present at any age but commonly occur in the first two decades of life.
2. Spitzoid melanomas are malignant melanocytic proliferations that share architectural and cytomorphologic attributes with Spitz nevi.
3. Atypical spitzoid neoplasms (also termed atypical Spitz tumors) represent a controversial concept forwarded by some to categorize lesions that have architecture and cytomorphology of indefinite significance. The authors believe this designation should be used as a provisional diagnostic category rather than interpreted as an entity sui generis.
4. The biologic behavior of melanocytic lesions is judged by the assessment of architectural and cytologic attributes, including, importantly, an assessment of symmetry, circumscription, maturation, and cellular proliferation.
5. Differentiating Spitz nevi, atypical spitzoid neoplasms, and spitzoid melanoma requires precise microscopic evaluation coupled with clinicopathologic correlation.

concept of MELTUMP (Melanocytic Tumor of Unknown Malignant Potential) overlaps the spectrum of atypical spitzoid neoplasms and represents a histopathologic gray area. Whether atypical spitzoid neoplasms should be thought of as a distinct entity or as a hodgepodge of peculiar Spitz nevi and borderline spitzoid melanomas remains a matter of debate. The authors believe the latter possibility is most likely.

The term "malignant Spitz nevus" was used to categorize a collection of nodular spitzoid proliferations that developed in children, adolescents, and young adults. Extended follow-up demonstrated that secondary spread to lymph nodes occurred not uncommonly but that widespread metastatic dissemination was rare. The designation of malignant Spitz nevus represents an oxymoron and its use as a diagnostic term is not endorsed. The authors suspect that lesions within this spectrum hold low-grade malignant potential and should be considered distinct from conventional adult-type melanoma, and the authors have used the designation spitzoid melanoma of childhood/adolescence or childhood-type melanoma in this context. Others have included lesions of this type within the spectrum of atypical spitzoid neoplasms.

The key to precise classification of Spitz nevi, atypical spitzoid neoplasms, and spitzoid melanoma remains careful microscopic evaluation coupled with clinicopathologic correlation. Molecular assessment by comparative genomic hybridization (CGH) and fluorescence in situ hybridization (FISH) are increasingly being used to screen lesions for genomic anomalies known to be associated with melanoma.

GROSS FEATURES

Spitz nevi are commonly reported to have a lateral diameter of 6 mm or less but breadth of up to 3 cm has been documented. Lesions may be pink, red, brown, or black in color. Many Spitz nevi are soft upon palpation, although desmoplastic Spitz nevi are characteristically firm and dermatofibroma like in character. Often, an initial period of rapid growth is followed by stability in size. Solitary lesions are the rule, but multilesional or agminated presentations have been documented. Occasional Spitz nevi may be polypoid or verrucous in configuration. Pigmented Spitz nevi are sometimes referred to as pigmented spindle cell nevi or Reed's nevi. The eponym honors Richard Reed, who popularized the designation pigmented spindle cell nevus.

For purposes of this article, Spitz nevi and pigmented spindle cell nevi represent variations within a broad spectrum rather than independent entities.

Spitzoid melanomas commonly have a lateral diameter of greater than 6 mm, and lesional size often exceeds 1 cm. Although clinical morphology has not been precisely tabulated, spitzoid melanomas present as papules, plaques, or nodules. Varied pigmentation can be seen. The authors' experience is that many, if not most, lesions are amelanotic.

As a bridge or provisional diagnostic category, it is difficult to provide stereotypical clinical morphology of an atypical spitzoid neoplasm. Suffice it to say that the clinical appearance of an atypical spitzoid neoplasm, much like that of a spitzoid melanoma, is not distinctive.

MICROSCOPIC FEATURES

Spitz nevi can be junctional, compound, or wholly dermal.[4,5] They typically hold symmetric, dome-shaped or wedge-shaped, well-circumscribed low power architecture with sharp lateral demarcation, generally ending in a nest at the peripheral border. Associated epidermal hyperplasia, hypergranulosis, and hyperkeratosis are common. At the junction, Spitz nevi display nests of spindled or epithelioid cells with ample cytoplasm and monomorphous nuclei with open chromatin and uniform nucleoli. Pericellular clefts often separate individual melanocytes or nests from contiguous structures, especially the acanthotic background epidermis (**Fig. 1**). Kamino bodies, which are acellular structures composed of basement membrane material that assume a dull-pink globular appearance with scalloped borders, are often found within the epidermis above dermal papillae. Any subjacent dermal component matures with descent such that nests of

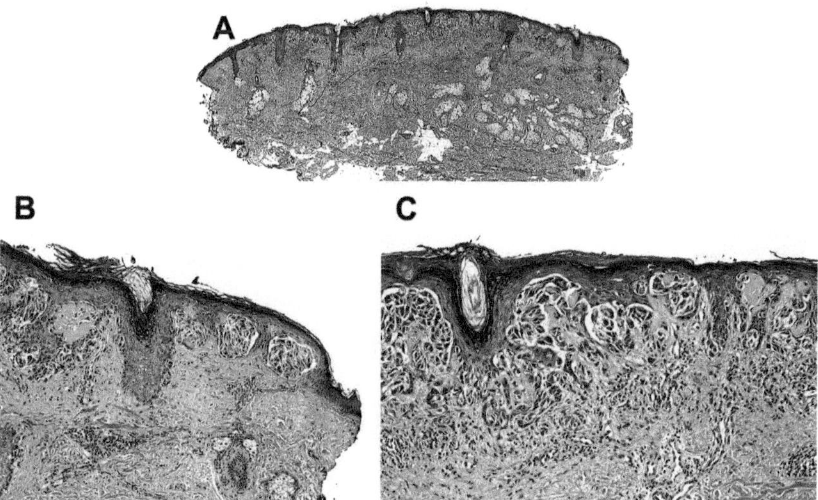

Fig. 1. Spitz nevus occurring within an adult. This complete excisional specimen shows good circumscription and a mostly nested configuration, despite the occurrence of the lesion within actinically damaged skin (*A*). Sharp circumscription is apparent at the lesion's edge (*B*). Centrally within the proliferation, large spindled and epithelioid melanocytes are separated from adjacent cells and structures by pericellular clefts, and many well-formed Kamino bodies are apparent above dermal papillae (*C*). Only small numbers of cells are scattered above the junction.

melanocytes become smaller and transition to individual melanocytes and encompassing dermal sclerosis (desmoplasia) is commonplace. Although occasional mitotic figures can be found within the epidermis and superficial dermis, there is characteristically a low dermal mitotic rate and any deep mitotic figures should be viewed with suspicion. Intraepidermal scatter (pagetoid spread) can be seen and in some instances is pronounced, but commonly suprabasal scatter is limited in degree and is limited in extent to the central portion of the lesion (**Fig. 2**).

Pigmented spindle cell nevi represent Spitz nevi with prominent cytoplasmic pigmentation. Lesions within the spectrum of pigmented spindle cell nevus are often composed of slender cells and a fascicular arrangement may be apparent along the junctional zone or in the upper dermis. Pigmented spindle cell nevi share many attributes in common with the broader spectrum of Spitz nevi, as they are often associated with acanthosis, hyperkeratosis, and well-formed Kamino bodies. The authors thus view pigmented spindle cell nevus as a variant within the broader spectrum of Spitz nevus rather than as an independent entity.

Spitzoid melanomas represent melanomas that hold architectural and cytologic resemblance to Spitz nevi (**Figs. 3** and **4**). As the determination of what is spitzoid and what is not is subjective, the designation is prone to overuse in the adult age group. As a generality, melanomas that display spindled or epithelioid cytomorphology and have associated epidermal hyperplasia are prone to be designated as spitzoid. Attributes favoring a diagnosis of spitzoid melanoma rather than Spitz nevus include a lack of symmetry, defective circumscription, epidermal and dermal confluence, and a lack of maturation with dermal descent. Additional worrisome findings include deep dermal mitotic figures, atypical mitotic figures, necrosis, and a lack of uniformity across lateral strata. Cytologically, high nuclear-to-cytoplasmic ratio, dusty

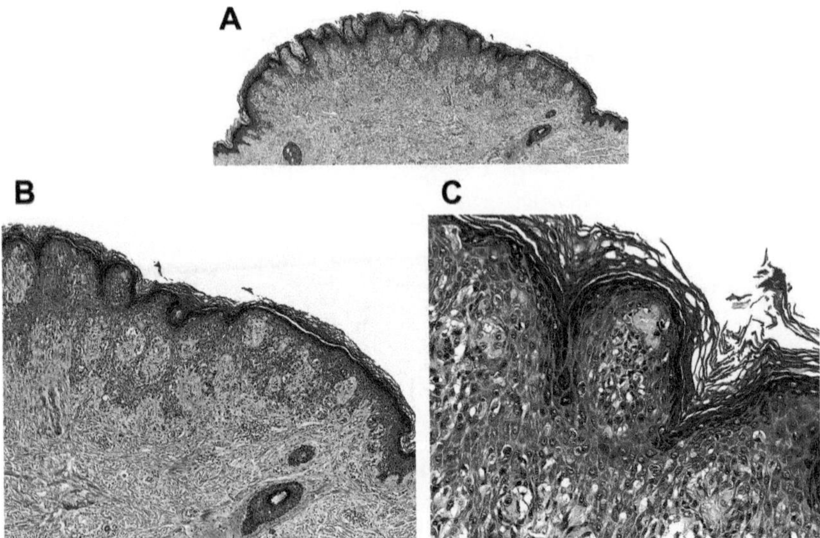

Fig. 2. Spitz nevus (with associated intraspinous scatter of cells) occurring on the knee. Small size and a mostly nested configuration are apparent at low magnification (*A*). The peripheral edge of the specimen shows reasonable lateral demarcation (*B*). At high magnification, many lesional cells are apparent in pagetoid array in the stratum spinosum (*C*). A well-formed Kamino body is also apparent. This degree of intraspinous scatter is not uncommon in volar Spitz nevi or in Spitz nevi from the knee or elbow.

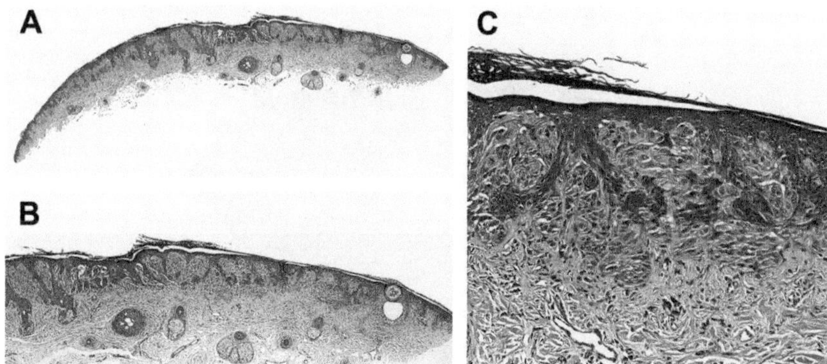

Fig. 3. Spitzoid melanoma occurring on the ear of a 35-year-old man. The lesion extends across the full breadth of the specimen and circumscription cannot be assessed (*A*). Large spindled and epithelioid melanocytes with fine cytoplasmic pigmentation are arrayed confluently along the junctional zone in concert with epithelial hyperplasia and orthohyperkeratosis (*B*). With high magnification scrutiny, Kamino bodies cannot be found (*C*). Fluorescence in situ hybridization analysis demonstrate chromosome 6p gain and an imbalance in chromosome 6q, favoring classification as spitzoid melanoma.

cytoplasmic melanization, and large eosinophilic nucleoli favor classification as melanoma.

As a provisional or bridge categorization, it is impossible to precisely define the histopathological criteria for an atypical spitzoid neoplasm (**Fig. 5**). The term "atypical Spitz nevus" was first used by Reed and colleagues[6] in 1975 to describe a spitzoid lesion that had densely cellular fascicles of spindled cells that compressed its stroma. It has subsequently been used to describe lesions of large size (>1 cm) with dense

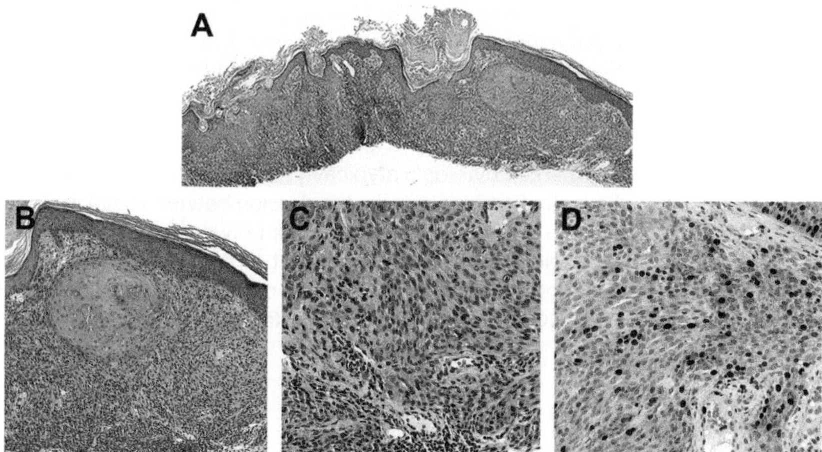

Fig. 4. Childhood-type spitzoid melanoma occurring on the buttock of a 17-year-old boy. This lesion shows reasonable circumscription and is associated with verrucous acanthosis, much like a Spitz nevus (*A*). However, in contrast to the configuration of a classical Spitz nevus, this proliferation is composed of large fascicles of nonmaturing spindled melanocytes (*B*). Dermal melanocytes in mitosis are easily found, including a mitosis centrally within this frame (*C*). A high–Ki-67 index is also apparent in this lesion (*D*).

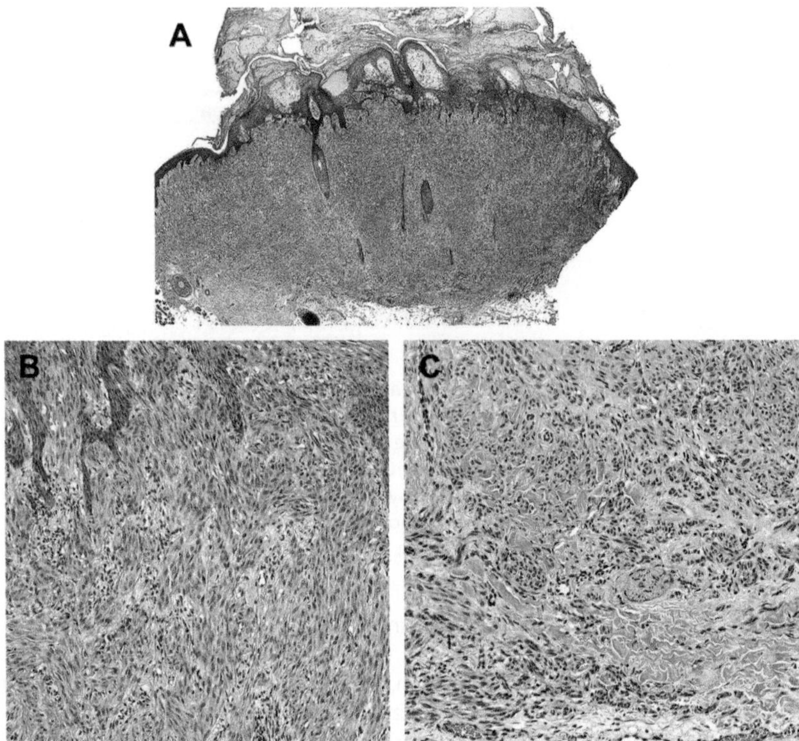

Fig. 5. Compound spitzoid neoplasm from the ear of a 5-year-old boy. This hypercellular lesion clinically resembled a keratoacanthoma. A sizable primary excision revealed a cellular proliferation of large spindled melanocytes that reached from the junctional zone to the superficial subcutis (*A*). Circumscription could not be assessed. Large fascicles of melanocytes are apparent along the junctional zone (*B*), and subjacent, deep dermal lesional melanocytes are similar and lack full maturation (*C*). Fluoresvcence in situ hybridization analysis demonstrated no aberrations. A re-excision specimen revealed no residuum. Classification as a hypercellular Spitz nevus was favored.

cellularity, deep extension, marked cytologic atypicality, increased mitoses, and associated ulceration. With the lack of precise criteria, the division between what is a peculiar but benign Spitz nevus and an atypical Spitz nevus, or between what is an atypical spitzoid neoplasm and spitzoid melanoma, may vary at different centers or among different interpreters. It is hoped that the development of fastidious histopathologic criteria and increased use of CGH and FISH analysis will facilitate diagnostic precision in this area.

DIFFERENTIAL DIAGNOSIS

The primary differential for spitzoid melanocytic lesions involves the distinction of a Spitz nevus from spitzoid melanoma. As no single attribute is sufficiently specific, the constellation of attributes listed in the Differential Diagnosis box should be coupled with an assessment of the clinical context. Prototypically, a small circumscribed lesion that matures with descent occurring in a child is readily interpreted as a Spitz nevus by the pathologist or dermatopathologist who is sufficiently knowledgeable and

Differential Diagnosis
Attributes utilized to differentiate Spitz nevi and Spitzoid melanoma

Favoring Benignancy	Of Concern for Melanoma
Symmetric, typically; modest asymmetry can be overlooked	Asymmetry
Crisply circumscribed, classically; minor defects in circumscription may occur, especially in lesions with associated suprabasal scatter	Poor circumscription, although a sharp lateral border can occasionally be found
Matures with descent: nests and cells become smaller with increasing dermal depth	Lacks maturation; a lack of maturation coupled with dermal melanocytes in mitosis provokes special worry
Large and well-formed Kamino bodies, or the presence of many small, well-formed Kamino bodies	Lacks Kamino bodies, or the Kamino bodies present are small and poorly formed
Prominent pericellular clefts, either around individual cells or around perijunctional nests	Lacks pericellular clefts
Limited intraepidermal (pagetoid) scatter	Florid intraepidermal scatter
Limited dermal proliferation (few detectable dermal mitoses)	Accentuated dermal proliferation (with readily detectable dermal mitoses)
Although enlarged, nuclei show little pleomorphism and have regular nuclear membranes and ground-glass cytoplasm	Pronounced nuclear pleomorphism, especially if coupled with fine dusty cytoplasmic melanization
Necrosis absent	Necrosis, either as single cells or en masse
Variable in size, often small	Variable in size, often large
Confined to the junction and upper reticular dermis	Deep reticular dermal or bulbous subcutaneous extension
Prominent epidermal hyperplasia with hypergranulosis and hyperkeratosis	Consumption of the epidermis, with diminishment of epithelial thickness and muting of rete

experienced (**Fig. 6**). Conversely, a large, asymmetrical, poorly circumscribed spitzoid lesion with many associated deep mitotic figures is easily classified as spitzoid melanoma. The challenge falls in the spectrum between these two poles. It remains clear that there are lesions for which an unequivocal diagnosis is extremely difficult, if not impossible.

The authors believe that the able distinction of a Spitz nevus from melanoma is best made with well-prepared sections by an experienced interpreter, which is particularly true if the case in question is challenging. Use of an expert consultant can be helpful in this context. Many problematic consultation cases can be solved simply by obtaining level sections or by obtaining a good quality recut section. The desire to obtain deeper sections should be balanced with the need to preserve tissue for possible molecular analysis by way of CGH and FISH.

Immunohistochemical evaluation of spitzoid lesions has, for the most part, not been proven to be of value in differential diagnosis. Spitz nevi and spitzoid melanomas often display diffuse expression of S-100 protein and Melan-A (MART-1). HMB-45, in contrast, demonstrates diminished expression toward the base of Spitz nevi. However, in the authors' experience this has not proven to be of clear diagnostic

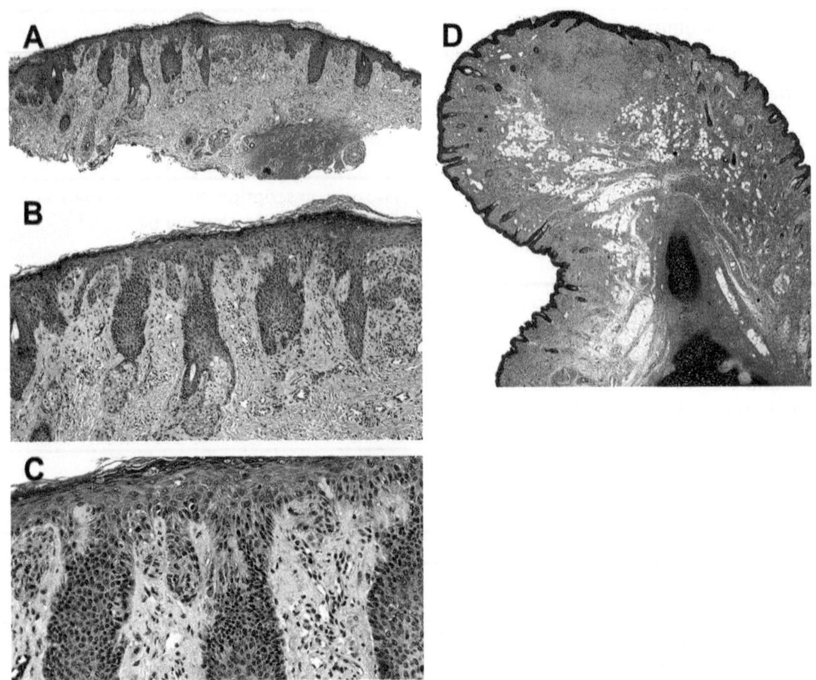

Fig. 6. Spitz nevus misdiagnosed as melanoma from the ear of a young adult. A mostly nested proliferation with large nests of enlarged melanocytes are apparent at scanning magnification (*A*), and closer inspection reveals incomplete maturation of nests in the dermis (*B*). At high magnification, a lack of suprabasal scatter and well-formed Kamino bodies are apparent (*C*). The errant diagnosis of melanoma triggered a sizable re-excision (*D*) with cosmetic implications (no residuum is found in the re-excision specimen).

value, as diminished HMB-45 expression can also be found in association with many melanomas. The primary immunoperoxidase analysis of value represents assessment of cell proliferation using markers, such as Ki-67. Kapor and colleagues[7] have shown Ki-67 labeling indices of 0.5% in conventional melanocytic nevi, 5% in conventional Spitz nevi, 10% in atypical spitzoid neoplasms, and nearly 40% in conventional melanomas. In short, a high–Ki-67 labeling rate in the assessment of a spitzoid lesion represents a cause for concern. It is important to keep in mind that a low labeling rate does not exclude melanoma, as the authors have encountered many melanomas with low–Ki-67 expression.

CGH and FISH represent methods used to determine DNA copy number changes that have been associated with certain types of melanocytic lesions and represent promising new methods for assessment of proliferations with ambiguous biologic potential. CGH of most Spitz nevi reveals no genomic aberrations, whereas 20% to 25% of Spitz nevi harbor an isolated gain of chromosome 11p, an anomaly that has not been documented in association with melanoma.[8] In contrast, over 95% of melanomas harbor multiple chromosomal aberrations, including gains and losses.[9,10] The advantage of CGH is that the entire genome is analyzed, but the complexity of the assay restricts its application to specialized centers. In contrast, FISH represents a more expeditious technique that should be broadly applicable using a probe set targeting specific loci of interest that have been defined from CGH data sets. At present, the authors are using a probe set analyzing loci on chromosomes 6p, 6q, 6centromere, and 11q, and this probe combination holds 85% sensitivity for detection of melanoma-associated genomic anomalies.[11] One concern is that the currently used probe set may hold lower sensitivity for the detection of childhood-type spitzoid melanoma in comparison with conventional (adult-type) melanoma, and probe sets tailored to specific differential diagnostic situations are currently under development.

PROGNOSIS

Classical Spitz nevi represent benign melanocytic lesions that hold no potential for metastasis and uncommonly persist after incomplete removal. Spitz nevi tend not to persist at the biopsy site if a given lesion was interpreted clinically to be removed, even if the margin was positive histopathologically.[12]

The prognosis of spitzoid melanoma is difficult to ascertain from the literature as current data includes heterogeneous patient populations. The authors suspect that older patients who have spitzoid melanoma hold a prognosis similar to that of other adult-type melanomas of similar thickness. In contrast, the authors suspect that the terms malignant Spitz nevus, spitzoid melanoma of childhood/adolescence, and childhood-type spitzoid melanoma represent similar if not identical lesions with low-grade malignant potential, including the potential for nodal spread, as indicated by the common finding of sentinel lymph node positivity. However, the authors suspect that such lesions hold much lower potential for the seeding of widespread distant metastases in comparison with conventional adult melanoma. Clearly, additional long-term studies, perhaps stratified by molecular results, are required to more clearly define prognosis in this context.

Lesions that have been classified as atypical spitzoid neoplasms have been associated with sentinel lymph node positivity; however, completion lymphadenectomy has typically revealed no additional nodal positivity and 2- to 3-year follow-ups have shown no further disease recurrence.[13,14] As expressed previously, the authors remain concerned that in the absence of precise diagnostic criteria, such information cannot be properly interpreted if lesions classified as atypical spitzoid neoplasms represent a heterogeneous grouping (of peculiar Spitz nevi and spitzoid melanomas). If a given lesion is classified as an atypical spitzoid neoplasm at one center and as a childhood-type melanoma at another, differences in data between the two centers will prove to be impossible to reconcile.

Although there is no broad consensus regarding the management of Spitz nevi and atypical spitzoid neoplasms, the authors offer the following general comments:

The authors routinely recommend conservative complete re-excision of the vast majority of spitzoid lesions that the authors believe to be classical Spitz nevi if they

Pitfalls
Spitz nevi and melanoma

! A partial biopsy of a larger melanocytic lesion, which prevents an assessment of size and lateral demarcation, can trigger an erroneous benign interpretation in the assessment of a melanoma, particularly if the melanoma is mostly nested in its distribution or spitzoid in its cytomorphology.

! Intraepidermal (pagetoid) scatter associated with an otherwise conventional Spitz nevus can elicit an incorrect diagnosis of (spitzoid) melanoma.

! A diagnosis of Spitz nevus should be made with caution in patients more than 50 years old.

display peculiar or atypical features. This step is intended to ensure complete removal, to prevent persistence, and to enable definitive microscopic evaluation of the entire lesion.

For microscopically classical Spitz nevi that have been adequately sampled, the authors tend to favor close clinical monitoring over further surgery as a management strategy if margins are positive, particularly if patients are young or if general anesthesia would be required to permit re-excision.

All atypical spitzoid neoplasms require full excision, as this provisional designation indicates, by definition, a lesion of uncertain biologic potential.

All patients should be managed on an individual basis to avoid undertreatment or overtreatment of these intriguing lesions.

REFERENCES

1. Herreid P, Shapiro P. Age distribution of Spitz nevus vs malignant melanoma. Arch Dermatol 1996;132:352–3.
2. Ackerman A. Spitz nevus. Am J Dermatopathol 1997;19(4):419–21.
3. Barnhill R, Argenyi Z, From L, et al. Atypical Spitz nevi/tumors: lack of consensus for diagnosis, discrimination from melanoma, and prediction of outcome. Hum Pathol 1999;30(5):513–20.
4. Massi G, LeBoit P. Histological diagnosis of nevi and melanoma. Germany: Steinkopff Verlag Darmstadt; 2004.
5. Barnhill R. The spitzoid lesion: rethinking Spitz tumors, atypical variants, 'Spitzoid' melanoma and risk assessment. Mod Pathol 2006;19:S21–33.
6. Reed R, Ichinose H, Clark W, et al. Common and uncommon melanocytic nevi and borderline melanomas. Semin Oncol 1975;2:119–47.
7. Kapor P, Selim M, Roy L, et al. Spitz nevi and atypical Spitz nevi/tumors: a histologic and immunohistochemical analysis. Mod Pathol 2005;18:197–204.
8. Bastian B, Wesselmann U, Pinkel D, et al. Molecular cytogenetic analysis of Spitz nevi shows clear differentiation to melanoma. J Invest Dermatol 1999;113: 1065–9.
9. Bastian B, LeBoit P, Hamm H, et al. Chromosomal gains and losses in primary cutaneous melanomas detected by comparative genomic hybridization. Cancer Res 1998;58:2170–5.
10. Curtin J, Fridlyand J, Kageshita T, et al. Distinct sets of genetic alterations in melanoma. N Engl J Med 2005;353:2135–47.
11. Gerami P, Jewell S, Morrison L, et al. Fluorescence in situ hybridization (FISH) as an ancillary diagnostic tool in the diagnosis of melanoma. Am J Surg Pathol 2009; 33(8):1146–56.
12. Kaye V, Deher L. Spindle and epithelioid cell nevus (Spitz nevus). Natural history following biopsy. Arch Dermatol 1990;126:1581–3.
13. Su L, Fullen D, Sondak V, et al. Sentinel lymph node biopsy for patients with problematic spitzoid melanocytic lesions: a report on 18 patients. Cancer 2003;97: 499–507.
14. Roaten J, Patrick D, Pearlman N, et al. Sentinel lymph node biopsy for melanoma and other melanocytic tumors in adolescents. J Pediatr Surg 2005;40:232–5.

Desmoplastic Melanoma

Klaus J. Busam, MD[a,b,*]

KEYWORDS

- Desmoplastic melanoma • Desmoplastic nevus
- Melanoma diagnosis • Sarcomatoid skin tumors • Prognosis

DESMOPLASTIC MELANOMA

Overview

Desmoplastic melanoma is characterized by the association of invasive melanoma with a prominent stromal fibrosis. Conley, Orr, and Lattes introduced the term desmoplastic melanoma (DM) in 1971, describing a "variant of spindle cell melanoma which produces or elicits the production of abundant collagen."[1] In the words of Reed and Leonard,[2] DM are "fibrous tumors whose individual spindle cells are isolated in a dense fibrous matrix."

Desmoplastic melanoma is uncommon, representing less than 4% of melanomas seen at large cancer centers.[3] Familiarity with DM is relevant for clinicians and pathologists because, for the unwary, this tumor may represent a diagnostic pitfall and lead to confusion with benign lesions, including fibrosing tumors and scars.[4]

Key Features
Desmoplastic melanoma

Extent of intratumoral fibrosis

May be prominent throughout the entire tumor (pure DM)

May represent a portion of an otherwise nondesmoplastic melanoma (combined DM)

Most often affects the head and neck region, but can occur anywhere, including acral and mucosal sites. Classic DM presents as a pauci-cellular scar like tumor.

A version of this article was previously published in *Surgical Pathology Clinics* 2:3.
[a] Department of Pathology, Memorial Sloan-Kettering Cancer Center, 1275 York Avenue, New York, NY 10021, USA
[b] Weill Medical College of Cornell University, New York, NY, USA
* Department of Pathology, Memorial Sloan-Kettering Cancer Center, 1275 York Avenue, New York, NY 10021.
E-mail address: busamk@mskcc.org

Clin Lab Med 31 (2011) 321–330
doi:10.1016/j.cll.2011.03.009 **labmed.theclinics.com**

Clinical Features

Desmoplastic melanoma is most commonly found on chronically sun-damaged skin of elderly individuals (men more often than women), but may also affect younger patients.[5–8] The male to female ratio is approximately 1.7:1. The median age at diagnosis of DM is approximately 10 years later than for conventional melanoma. This difference is likely related to delays in diagnosis (DM is more difficult to recognize clinically in its early stage than conventional melanoma) and an inherent difference in the biology of the lesion (association of DM with lentigo maligna and chronic sun damage). DM most often affects the head and neck region, but it can occur anywhere, including acral and mucosal sites.[5–10] In the United States, approximately 20% of DM are found on the torso, 20% on the extremities, and the rest on the head and neck.

DM usually presents as a firm papule, nodule or plaque. It is often associated with a lentigo maligna, which is why it is advisable to palpate the skin overlying or surrounding a lentigo maligna, or excision sites thereof, to better detect a dermal tumor. However, DM may develop in the absence of a clinically detectable precursor lesion. Pigmentation is often lacking, but shades of tan or erythema may be present. Because of the lack of characteristic clinical features, correct identification of DM by a clinician is uncommon and the tumor is rarely diagnosed at an early stage.[11] The clinical impression of lesions that ultimately prove to be DM typically includes a scar, fibroma, or cyst. Seborrheic keratosis, eczema, or melanocytic nevus may also be considered. Occasionally, the differential diagnosis will include malignant lesions, such as basal cell carcinoma, squamous cell carcinoma, sarcoma, or amelanotic melanoma.

Microscopic Features

Most DM are fibrosing spindle cell tumors (**Figs. 1** and **2**). Rarely, an epithelioid cell melanoma shows prominent intratumoral fibrosis. Classic DM presents as a paucicellular, scar like tumor.[5] Because of the abundance of fibrous tissue, DM has a pink appearance at scanning magnification. Most DM display a diffusely infiltrative

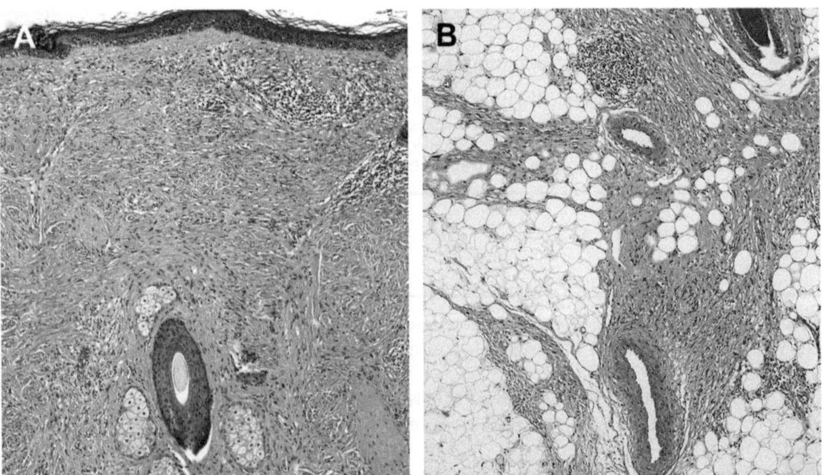

Fig. 1. Desmoplastic melanoma. (*A*) Infiltration of the dermis by spindle cells. (*B*) The malignant spindle cells diffusely infiltrate the subcutis and are associated with lymphocytic aggregates.

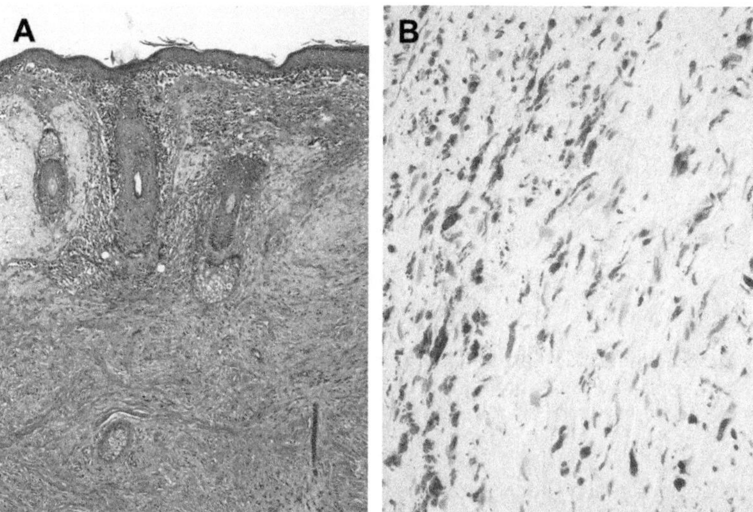

Fig. 2. Desmoplastic melanoma. (*A*) In situ melanoma is association with an invasive fibrosing spindle cell proliferation. (*B*) The spindle cell proliferation is immunoreactive for S-100 protein.

pattern with expansion of subcutaneous fibrous septa and eventual replacement of the fat lobules by tumor and its desmoplastic stroma. Lymphocytic aggregates are often present (see **Fig. 1**B). Superficially, an associated in situ melanoma component is identified in 80% to 85% of cases (see **Fig. 2**).[5,12] Perineural invasion is commonly seen, especially with thicker tumors in the head and neck region (**Fig. 3**).

Cytologic atypia of tumor cells in DM can be variable ranging from a fairly bland appearance to marked nuclear pleomorphism.[5] If the cytology is overall bland and the tumor cells have a fibroblast like appearance there is potential confusion with a scar. If the tumor cells differentiate along Schwannian lines, the features of the tumor cells may at times mimic the cells of a neurofibroma, neurotized melanocytic nevus, or nerve sheath myxoma. Bland cytology is rarely uniform throughout the entire tumor and poses a diagnostic problem usually only on partial biopsies. When DM is frankly

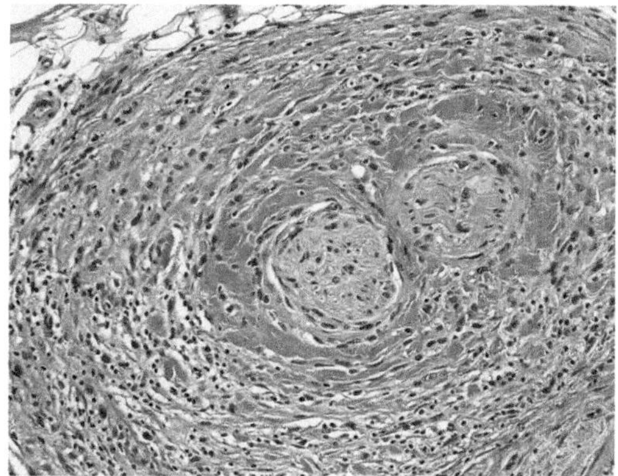

Fig. 3. Desmoplastic melanoma with perineural invasion.

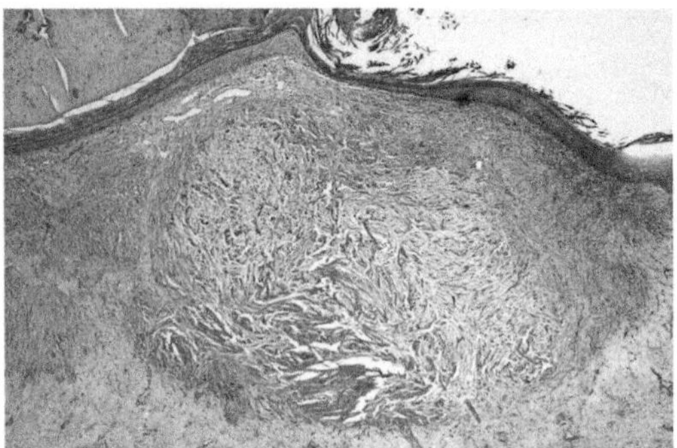

Fig. 4. Myxoid desmoplastic melanoma. Most of the tissue shows a pauci-cellular spindle cell proliferation associated with abundant collagen, but there are foci of dense aggregates of fusiform melanocytes, which are cytologically more atypical.

pleomorphic, it is readily recognized as malignant, but in the absence of melanin pigment and in situ melanoma, may be confused with a sarcoma or sarcomatoid carcinoma.

A subset of DM has a myxoid material (**Fig. 4**),[13–15] which may lead to potential confusion with other myxoid soft-tissue tumors (especially of fibrous or nerve sheath origin)[16] or sclerosing mucinous melanocytic nevi.[17]

DESMOPLASTIC MELANOMA VERSUS A SCLEROSING MELANOCYTIC NEVUS

Differential Diagnosis

Desmoplasia may also be associated with benign melanocytic nevi, such as pauci- or amelanotic-sclerosing variants of blue nevus, Spitz nevus, or other nevi,[17]and lead to potential confusion with DM (**Table 1**).

Differential Diagnosis
Desmoplastic melanoma

Benign lesions

- Sclerosing melanocytic nevus
- Dermal scar
- Dermatofibroma
- Neurofibroma
- Pleomorphic fibroma

Malignant tumors

- Sarcomatoid carcinoma
  - Sclerosing spindle cell squamous cell carcinoma
- Sarcoma
  - Spindle cell sarcoma (fibrosarcoma, myxofibrosarcoma)
  - Leiomyosarcoma
  - Malignant Peripheral Nerve Sheath Tumor (MPNST)

Table 1
Desmoplastic melanoma versus desmoplastic melanocytic nevus

	Desmoplastic Melanoma	Desmoplastic Nevus
Silhouette	Asymmetric	Symmetric
Growth pattern	Irregular and infiltrative	Circumscribed (orderly)
Maturation	Absent	Present
Atypia	Usually present; often moderate	Usually absent, except for sclerosing Spitz's nevi
Mitoses	Common	Usually absent
In situ melanoma	Often present	Absent
Junctional nevus	Absent	May be present
Lymphocytic aggregates	Common	Rare
Replacement of fat	Common	Absent, except for congenital nevi with sclerosis
Immunophenotype	Usually negative, rarely positive for MDA	Usually positive for MDA

Abbreviation: MDA, melanocytic differentiation antigens (Melan-A/Mart-1, tyrosinase, gp100, microphthalmia transcription factor).

Sclerosing nevi often occur in patients younger than the average age of diagnosis for DM and are less commonly found in markedly sun-damaged skin.[18–20] Histologically, they display a benign circumscribed silhouette. Cytologic atypia and mitotic figures are usually absent. In contrast, DM tend to be asymmetric, infiltrative, and poorly circumscribed. The majority of DM is associated with in situ melanoma. If a sclerosing nevus has a junctional melanocytic proliferation, it has features of a benign nevus.

Immunohistochemistry can be helpful for the distinction of sclerosing nevus from melanoma.[21] Most sclerosing nevi are immunoreactive for Melan-A or other differentiation markers, while DM tend to be negative.

DESMOPLASTIC MELANOMA VERSUS A NONMELANOCYTIC SPINDLE CELL PROLIFERATION

Distinction from Dermal Scar or Fibroma

In the absence of associated intraepidermal melanoma, recognition of a dermal spindle cell tumor as melanoma can be difficult. DM may be mistaken for a scar[22,23] or fibroma.[19] Scars are best distinguished from invasive DM by examining the growth pattern of the spindle cells, their cytology, and by analysis of associated features, such as vascularity. In scars, the fibroblasts are typically oriented parallel to the skin surface, while the blood vessels often run perpendicular to it. In dermatofibromas, the spindle cells tend to wrap around collagen bundles. In DM, the spindle cells are often oriented vertically or diagonally to the surface. DM frequently displays some degree of nuclear atypia, most often in the form of elongated hyperchromatic nuclei. Lymphocytic aggregates are an important diagnostic clue. A fibrosing spindle cell proliferation with clusters of lymphocytes needs to be suspected to be a possible DM, keeping in mind that occasionally lymphoid aggregates can also be seen with a scar or fibroma.

If a distinction of a scar or fibroma by morphologic criteria is difficult (eg, pleomorphic fibroma vs DM), immunohistochemistry should clarify the diagnosis. Although scars and fibromas may contain scattered isolated S-100 protein-positive cells, they are typically negative for S-100 protein. In contrast, DM is typically strongly and diffusely positive for S-100 protein (see **Fig. 2**).[24,25]

Distinction from Sarcoma or Sarcomatoid Carcinoma

Pleomorphic variants of DM need to be distinguished from fibrosarcoma, desmoplastic leiomyosarcoma, and sclerosing sarcomatoid squamous cell carcinoma (**Table 2**).[5,26,27] Immunohistochemical studies are critical in this regard. A sensitive marker for the diagnosis of sarcomatoid carcinoma is the 34BE12, which usually does not stain melanomas. The distinction from fibrosarcoma or leiomyosarcoma rarely poses a challenge, because these tumors are usually negative for S-100 protein. However, caution must be used in interpreting immunostains for CD34, CD10, smooth muscle actin, or desmin because DM may stain with any of these markers.[28,29] DM can be difficult to distinguish from a malignant peripheral nerve sheath tumor (MPNST). MPNST is more cellular and often associated with a neurofibroma. Melanomas tend to be diffusely and strongly positive for S-100 protein, while MPNST usually only stain focally, but there are exceptions. Clinical and histologic context are important. For example, if a malignant spindle cell tumor occurs in patients who have neurofibromatosis, or in association with neurofibroma, the diagnosis of MPNST is straightforward.

Diagnosis

A diagnosis of DM can readily be established if an in situ melanoma component is associated with a fibrosing malignant spindle cell tumor. In the absence of a detectable in situ melanoma, strong diffuse immunoreactivity of the malignant dermal spindle cell tumor for S-100 protein (and lack of staining for epithelial markers) supports the diagnosis. Immunohistochemistry for the melanocyte differentiation antigens Melan-A, tyrosinase, HMB45, or microphthalmia transcription factor is usually negative in DM.[24,25] If the staining for S-100 protein is weak, labeling for nerve growth factor receptor (NGF-R) may be helpful.[30]

Because of the prominent fibrous stroma separating the tumor cells, the typical DM is overall pauci-cellular throughout the entire lesion. Small foci of higher cell density are not uncommon, but usually constitute a minor component of the tumor. In some

Table 2
Distinction of desmoplastic melanoma from sarcoma and sarcomatoid carcinoma

Marker	S-100 Protein	Muscle Markers	Epithelial Markers
Melanoma	Diffusely Positive	Usually negative, but may be positive for SMA or desmin	May be focally positive
Desmoplastic carcinoma	Usually negative	Usually negative, may be focally positive	Positive (34BE12, MNF116, p63, CK5/6)
Leiomyosarcoma	Negative	Positive	Negative
Pleomorphic sarcoma (MFH)	Usually negative	May be positive for SMA	Usually negative
MPNST	Often positive, usually focal	May be positive	Usually negative

Abbreviations: MFH, so-called "malignant fibrous histiocytoma"; MPNST, malignant peripheral nerve sheath tumor; SMA, smooth muscle actin.

tumors, dense cellular aggregates without any or much intratumoral fibrosis may dominate the picture of the invasive melanoma. There is no consensus as to the extent to which typical (ie, pauci-cellular fibrosing) features of DM need to be present for a tumor to qualify as DM. Most series of DM fail to precisely define the histologic criteria necessary for a diagnosis of DM. Recent data from Memorial Sloan-Kettering Cancer Center have highlighted the importance of strict criteria for DM.[5,8] A separation of pure from combined or mixed forms of DM was proposed. Pure DM were defined as melanomas in which 90% of the invasive tumor was desmoplastic with a pauci-cellular fibrosing appearance.[5,8] In combined DM, typical features of DM are mixed with dense cellular tumor foci without fibrosis. Several subsequent studies have supported the value of distinguishing pure from mixed tumors; pure DM tend to have a much lower incidence of positive sentinel lymph node (SLN) than mixed tumors (see later discussion).[31,32]

A subset of DM shows neurotropism. Reed and Leonard first brought attention to a group of melanomas characterized by neuroma like growth patterns and prominent infiltration of peripheral nerves (see **Fig. 3**).[2] They designated neurotropic melanoma (NM) as a variant of DM, classifying them as desmoplastic neurotropic melanomas (DNM).[3] However, it needs to be emphasized that not all neurotropic melanomas are desmoplastic. Many of them would fall into the category of mixed DM.

Additional subtypes of DNM have been described. In one variant, the invasive component closely simulates the growth pattern and cytologic appearance of a nerve sheath tumor (neurofibroma, if cytologically bland or neurosarcoma/malignant peripheral nerve sheath tumor, if the cytologic features are pleomorphic). This phenomenon has been described as so-called "neural transformation."[33,34] In another rare variant, the tumor is totally neurotropic in the sense that it is entirely confined to within the nerve and nerve sheath, leading to grossly visible nerve enlargement and thereby mimicking a primary nerve sheath tumor. This latter form of DNM has been termed "nerve-centered" DM.[33]

Prognosis

There is controversy with regard to the prognosis of DM.[8] In Conley and colleagues's[1] series of melanomas with desmoplasia, the tumors were described as "highly malignant stubbornly recurring and often metastasizing neoplasms." This characterization has contributed to the perception in the years thereafter that DM may be associated with worse clinical outcome than melanomas of the more usual type.

The perception of DM began to change in 1988 when Walsh and colleagues[35] suggested that DM may be associated with a more favorable outcome. The majority of subsequent studies supported this notion by reporting longer survival of patients who had DM compared with those who had conventional melanomas of similar thickness,[6,12,36] but the verdict was not unanimous.[3,37] The failure of some studies to detect differences between DM and conventional melanoma[3,37] may be, in part, attributable to the fact that they contained many more thin or intermediate thickness DM than others. The favorable prognostic impact of desmoplasia is best appreciated in deeply infiltrating melanomas, when additional Breslow thickness above and beyond 4 mm looses its prognostic strength. This hypothesis is supported by a study by Spatz and colleagues[38] who compared the histologic features of thick (>5 mm) melanomas from patients who had at least a 10-year survival with control cases of patients who died within 3 years of diagnosis. Seven of 42 subjects who had long-term survival had a DM. None of the thick tumors from 42 subjects who had short-term survival was desmoplastic.[38]

Pitfalls
Desmoplastic melanoma

! Rarity of occurrence presents a diagnostic pitfall and leads to confusion with benign lesions.

! DM May develop in the absence of a clinically detectable precursor lesion.

! Can be confused with a scar if cytology is bland and tumor cells have a fibroblast like appearance. Bland cytology is rarely uniform throughout the entire tumor and presents a diagnostic problem only on partial biopsies.

Another reason for conflicting results in the literature about clinical behavior of DM is heterogeneity among melanomas classified as desmoplastic.[8] Some reports suggest that the participating pathologists included tumors with variable degrees of desmoplasia, even if stromal fibrosis involved only a partial component of an otherwise conventional melanoma (equivalent to the term mixed or combined DM used herein).[8]

There is emerging consensus, however, from most melanoma programs, that DM is associated with a lower incidence of positive SLN than conventional melanomas. The difference is most striking if strict criteria are applied for the diagnosis of DM (ie, pure DM are less likely to metastasize to the regional node than mixed DM).[31,32,39–41]

REFERENCES

1. Conley J, Lattes R, Orr W. Desmoplastic malignant melanoma (a rare variant of spindle cell melanoma). Cancer 1971;28:914–36.
2. Reed RJ, Leonard DD. Neurotropic melanoma. A variant of desmoplastic melanoma. Am J Surg Pathol 1979;3:301–11.
3. Quinn MJ, Crotty KA, Thompson JF, et al. Desmoplastic and desmoplastic neurotropic melanoma: experience with 280 patients. Cancer 1998;83:1128–35.
4. McCarthy SW, Scolyer RA, Palmer AA. Desmoplastic melanoma: a diagnostic trap for the unwary. Pathology 2004;36:445–51.
5. Busam KJ, Mujumdar U, Hummer AJ, et al. Cutaneous desmoplastic melanoma: reappraisal of morphologic heterogeneity and prognostic factors. Am J Surg Pathol 2004;28:1518–25.
6. Skelton HG, Smith KJ, Laskin WB, et al. Desmoplastic malignant melanoma. J Am Acad Dermatol 1995;32:717–25.
7. Hawkins WG, Busam KJ, Ben-Porat L, et al. Desmoplastic melanoma: a pathologically and clinically distinct form of cutaneous melanoma. Ann Surg Oncol 2005; 12:207–13.
8. Chen JY, Hruby G, Scolyer RA, et al. Desmoplastic neurotropic melanoma: a clinicopathologic analysis of 128 cases. Cancer 2008;113:2770–8.
9. Su LD, Fullen DR, Lowe L, et al. Desmoplastic and neurotropic melanoma. Cancer 2004;100:598–604.
10. Kilpatrick SE, White WL, Browne JD. Desmoplastic malignant melanoma of the oral mucosa. An underrecognized diagnostic pitfall. Cancer 1996;78:383–9.
11. Wharton JM, Carlson JA, Mihm MC Jr. Desmoplastic malignant melanoma: diagnosis of early clinical lesions. Hum Pathol 1999;30:537–42.
12. Carlson JA, Dickersin GR, Sober AJ, et al. Desmoplastic neurotropic melanoma. A clinicopathologic analysis of 28 cases. Cancer 1995;75:478–94.
13. Sarode VR, Joshi K, Ravichandran P, et al. Myxoid variant of primary cutaneous malignant melanoma. Histopathology 1992;20:186–7.

14. Patel P, Levin K, Waltz K, et al. Myxoid melanoma: immunohistochemical studies and a review of the literature. J Am Acad Dermatol 2002;46:264–70.
15. Hitchcock MG, McCalmont TH, White WL. Cutaneous melanoma with myxoid features: twelve cases with differential diagnosis. Am J Surg Pathol 1999;23: 1506–13.
16. Allen PW. Myxoid tumors of soft tissues. Pathol Annu 1980;15:133–92.
17. Rongioletti F, Innocenzi D. Sclerosing 'mucinous' blue naevus. Br J Dermatol 2003;148:1250–2.
18. Busam KJ, Barnhill RL. Dermal melanocytoses, blue nevi and related conditions. In: Busam KJ, editor. Pathology of melanocytic nevi and malignant melanoma. New York: Springer; 2004. p. 199–222.
19. Harris GR, Shea CR, Horenstein MG, et al. Desmoplastic (sclerotic) nevus: an underrecognized entity that resembles dermatofibroma and desmoplastic melanoma. Am J Surg Pathol 1999;23:786–94.
20. Liu J, Cohen PR, Farhood A. Hyalinizing Spitz nevus: spindle and epithelioid cell nevus with paucicellular collagenous stroma. Southampt Med J 2004;97:102–6.
21. Kucher C, Zhang PJ, Pasha T, et al. Expression of Melan-A and Ki-67 in desmoplastic melanoma and desmoplastic nevi. Am J Dermatopathol 2004;26:452–7.
22. Kaneishi NK, Cockerell CJ. Histologic differentiation of desmoplastic melanoma from cicatrices. Am J Dermatopathol 1998;20:128–34.
23. Spitz JL, Silvers DN. Desmoplastic melanoma (or is it merely cicatrix?) arising at the site of biopsy within a conventional melanoma: pitfalls in the diagnosis desmoplastic melanoma. Cutis 1995;55:40–4.
24. Busam KJ, Iversen K, Coplan KC, et al. Analysis of microphthalmia transcription factor expression in normal tissues and tumors, and comparison of its expression with S-100 protein, gp100, and tyrosinase in desmoplastic malignant melanoma. Am J Surg Pathol 2001;25:197–204.
25. Winnepenninckx V, De Vos R, Stas M, et al. New phenotypical and ultrastructural findings in spindle cell (desmoplastic/neurotropic) melanoma. Appl Immunohistochem Mol Morphol 2003;11:319–25.
26. Diaz-Cascajo C, Borghi S, Weyers W. Desmoplastic leiomyosarcoma of the skin. Am J Dermatopathol 2000;22:251–5.
27. Kane CL, Keehn CA, Smithberger E, et al. Histopathology of cutaneous squamous cell carcinoma and its variants. Semin Cutan Med Surg 2004;23:54–61.
28. Hoang MP, Selim MA, Bentley RC, et al. CD34 expression in desmoplastic melanoma. J Cutan Pathol 2001;28:508–12.
29. Riccioni L, Di Tommaso L, Collina G. Actin-rich desmoplastic malignant melanoma: report of three cases. Am J Dermatopathol 1999;21:537–41.
30. Kanik AB, Yaar M, Bhawan J. p75 nerve growth factor receptor staining helps identify desmoplastic and neurotropic melanoma. J Cutan Pathol 1996;23: 205–10.
31. Pawlik TM, Ross MI, Prieto VG, et al. Assessment of the role of sentinel lymph node biopsy for primary cutaneous desmoplastic melanoma. Cancer 2006;106: 900–6.
32. George E, McClain SE, Slingluff CL, et al. Subclassification of desmoplastic melanoma: pure and mixed variants have significantly different capacities for lymph node metastasis. J Cutan Pathol 2009;36:425–32.
33. Jain S, Allen PW. Desmoplastic malignant melanoma and its variants. A study of 45 cases. Am J Surg Pathol 1989;13:358–73.
34. Smithers BM, McLeod GR, Little JH. Desmoplastic melanoma: patterns of recurrence. World J Surg 1992;16:186–90.

35. Walsh NM, Roberts JT, Orr W, et al. Desmoplastic malignant melanoma. A clinicopathologic study of 14 cases. Arch Pathol Lab Med 1988;112:922–7.
36. Baer SC, Schultz D, Synnestvedt M, et al. Desmoplasia and neurotropism. Prognostic variables in patients with stage I melanoma. Cancer 1995;76:2242–7.
37. Livestro DP, Muzikansky A, Kaine EM, et al. Biology of desmoplastic melanoma: a case-control comparison with other melanomas. J Clin Oncol 2005;23:6739–46.
38. Spatz A, Shaw HM, Crotty KA, et al. Analysis of histopathological factors associated with prolonged survival of 10 years or more for patients with thick melanomas (>5 mm). Histopathology 1998;33:406–13.
39. Gyorki DE, Busam K, Panageas K, et al. Sentinel lymph node biopsy for patients with cutaneous desmoplastic melanoma. Ann Surg Oncol 2003;10:403–7.
40. Thelmo MC, Sagebiel RW, Treseler PA, et al. Evaluation of sentinel lymph node status in spindle cell melanomas. J Am Acad Dermatol 2001;44:451–5.
41. Jaroszewski DE, Pockaj BA, DiCaudo DJ, et al. The clinical behavior of desmoplastic melanoma. Am J Surg 2001;182:590–5.

Molecular Aspects of Melanoma

Philip D. Da Forno, MBChB, MD, FRCPath[a,*],
Gerald S. Saldanha, MBChB, PhD, FRCPath, MRCP[b]

KEYWORDS

- Molecular pathology • Signature changes in melanoma
- Carcinogenesis • Melanoma genetics • Cell signaling

OVERVIEW: MOLECULAR PATHOLOGY OF MELANOMA

Dysregulation of the normal pathways of cell physiology is fundamental to carcinogenesis. Characterizing the changes that occur to the genes within these pathways will enhance understanding of how cancers arise and how they progress to advanced cancers, and it ultimately may lead to improved prognostication and treatment. Carcinogenesis is a multistep process, and typically, in order for a cell to become malignant, 4 to 7 rate-limiting stochastic genomic events occur.[1] In most human cancers these events are incompletely characterized, and currently many crucial genetic changes are yet to be discovered. Malignant melanoma is one such example. A handful of "core" changes have been identified that make up a genetic signature that is common to most melanomas (**Fig. 1**), but beyond this, there are genetic changes that precede, accompany, or arise from the signature changes and account for the great phenotypic variation observed clinicopathologically. These "noncore" changes are also incompletely understood, but some potentially crucial mediators of melanoma development and progression have emerged. This discussion begins by describing signature changes in melanoma.

SIGNATURE CHANGES IN MELANOMA

NRAS, BRAF, and the Mitogen-Activated Protein Kinase Pathway

The ras-raf-mek-erk mitogen-activated protein kinase (MAPK) pathway is a signaling cascade that transmits signals from the cell surface to the nucleus through a series of intermediate cytoplasmic proteins. Activation of the pathway affects proliferation, differentiation, senescence, and apoptosis (**Fig. 2**). Activating mutations of the

A version of this article was previously published in *Surgical Pathology Clinics* 2:3.
[a] Department of Histopathology, University Hospitals of Leicester NHS Trust, Sandringham Building, Leicester Royal Infirmary, Leicester, LE1 5WW UK
[b] Department of Cancer Studies and Molecular Medicine, Robert Kilpatrick Clinical Sciences Building, Leicester Royal Infirmary, PO Box 65, Leicester, LE2 7LX UK
* Corresponding author.
E-mail address: pddf1@yahoo.co.uk

Clin Lab Med 31 (2011) 331–343
doi:10.1016/j.cll.2011.03.010 labmed.theclinics.com
0272-2712/11/$ – see front matter

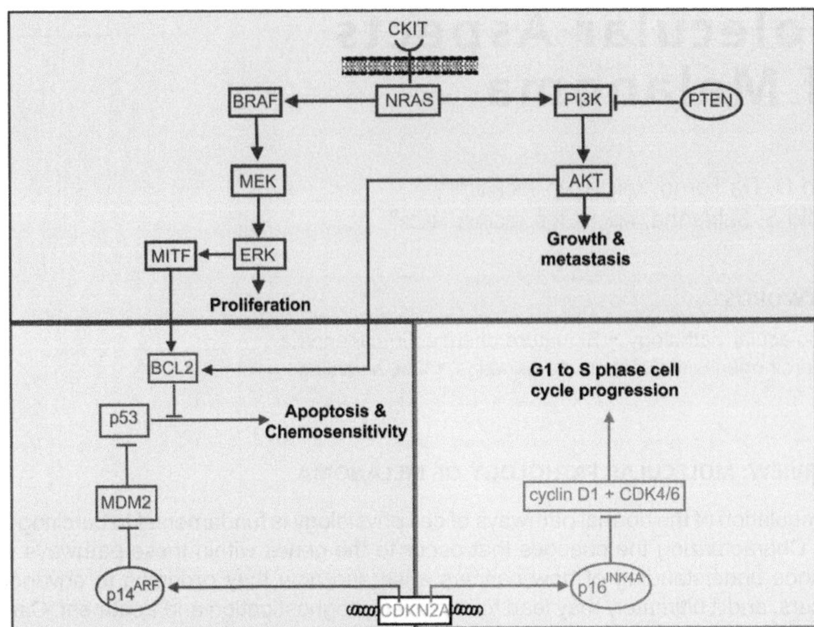

Fig. 1. Key signaling pathways in cutaneous malignant melanoma. The mitogen-activated protein kinase pathway (MAPK) and PTEN/PI3K pathways are shown in blue. The fundamental importance of CDKN2A is illustrated because it influences both the pRb (*shown in red*) and p53 pathways (*green*). In this simplified model, it can be seen that there is cross-talk between some of the pathways.

MAPK pathway enable cancer cells to become self-sufficient in growth signals, one of the hallmarks of cancer.[1]

The first MAPK alterations to be described in melanoma were oncogenic mutations of NRAS. Constitutive activation of ras uncouples the MAPK pathway from the need for external growth signals and consequently the pathway is continuously activated. The mutation frequency of NRAS in melanoma is approximately 20%,[2–5] whereas mutations of the other RAS genes, HRAS (11p15.5) and KRAS (12p12.1), are rare.[2,6]

The reported frequency of mutations of the downstream effector of ras, BRAF, varies but is typically reported to be between 50% and 70%.[4,6–10] More than 90% of the mutations of BRAF occur at codon 600[11] in exon 15, which increases its kinase activity by a factor of 500.[12] Despite exposure to UV radiation being the only known environmental risk factor for melanoma, the majority of BRAF mutations do not show the typical UV damage "signature" of transversions at pyrimidine dimers. Furthermore, BRAF mutations are not common in other skin cancer types whose incidence also correlates with 7UV radiation exposure, such as basal cell carcinoma.[13] This fact indicates that UV radiation does not directly damage the BRAF gene, but that the mutations occur via alternative mechanisms.[11]

Aside from melanoma, mutations of BRAF and NRAS are also described in up to 80% of nevi.[14–18] Many investigators have regarded this as evidence that mutations of BRAF and NRAS are early events in melanoma progression, because some melanomas are considered to arise within nevi.[19,20] Of note, Spitz nevi show a very low frequency of these mutations, although they do express high levels of proteins that lie downstream from ras and raf, such as erk.[18,21] The presence of BRAF and NRAS

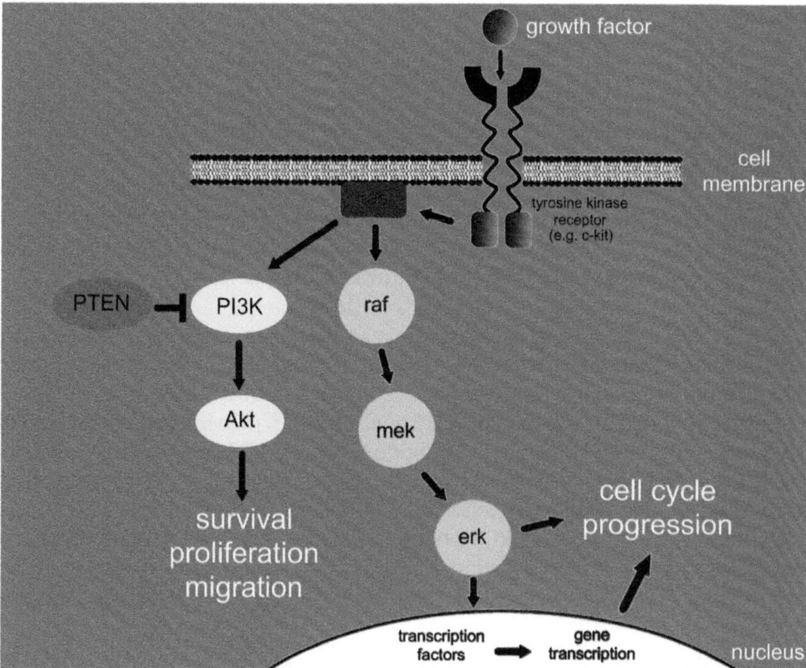

Fig. 2. The mitogen-activated protein kinase pathway (MAPK) and the ras-activated PTEN/PI3K pathway. Activating mutations of ras or PTEN loss with activating mutation of BRAF will negate the need for external growth signals to activate both pathways.

mutations in benign as well as malignant melanocytic tumors indicates that these alterations alone are not sufficient to cause malignancy, but may be important for the initiation of neoplasia.[17]

Mutations of NRAS and BRAF tend to be mutually exclusive in melanoma, a feature consistent with being effectors in the same pathway, and indicating the fundamental nature of MAPK pathway activation in melanoma development. There are, however, minor but notable exceptions to this rule, as described in the work of Curtin and colleagues and others.[22–25] Investigating RAS and RAF mutations has demonstrated the importance of activation of the MAPK and PI3K-Akt pathways. In many melanomas both of these pathways are activated either by simultaneous alterations of BRAF and PTEN, or by mutations of NRAS alone.[26,27] Alterations of the PI3K-Akt pathway, another signature change of melanoma, are now described.

PTEN and the PI3K Pathway

PTEN is a tumor suppressor gene that is mutated in up to 50% of melanoma cell lines and 20% of uncultured melanomas.[28] PTEN functions primarily by decreasing the activity of PI3K signaling (see **Fig. 2**), which results in arrested cell cycle progression and promotion of apoptosis. In the absence of functional PTEN, PI3K-Akt signaling is unchecked, producing upregulation of antiapoptotic proteins such as Bcl2, inhibition of the apoptotic protein bad, and transcription of cell cycle regulatory proteins. RAS activates both the PI3K and MAPK pathways, which again demonstrates the importance of RAS mutations in melanoma and indicates that PTEN and RAS have opposing functions in PI3K signaling. The former is a tumor suppressor and the latter oncogenic, a view supported by the reciprocal mutational status of PTEN and RAS observed in melanoma and other cancers.[26,27,29]

CDKN2A

The final signature change of melanoma to be described concerns the tumor suppressor gene CDK2NA, which is located on chromosome 9p21and encodes p16^{INK4a} and, via an alternate reading frame, p14^{ARF}. Mutation, methylation, and deletion of the CDKN2A gene is well described in both sporadic and familial melanomas, and is found in around 80% of cases.[30–34] Melanoma-associated CDKN2A mutations and deletions can involve p16^{INK4a}, p14^{ARF}, or both transcripts.

p16

p16^{INK4a} inhibits cyclin-dependent kinase 4 (cdk4) mediated hyperphosphorylation of the retinoblastoma protein (pRb), thereby ensuring the sequestration of E2F transcription factors (**Fig. 3**). In the absence of functional p16^{INK4a}, pRb is hyperphosphorylated via the actions of cdk4 and cyclin D, and consequently E2F transcription factors are released. E2F promotes the transcription of genes necessary for progression to S phase of the cell cycle. The G1-S checkpoint of the cell cycle is an important gateway to proliferation[35] because, once in S phase, cells are committed to replication.

There is loss of p16^{INK4a} expression as melanomas progress,[36–39] with the protein present in a significant number of radial growth phase and some vertical growth phase

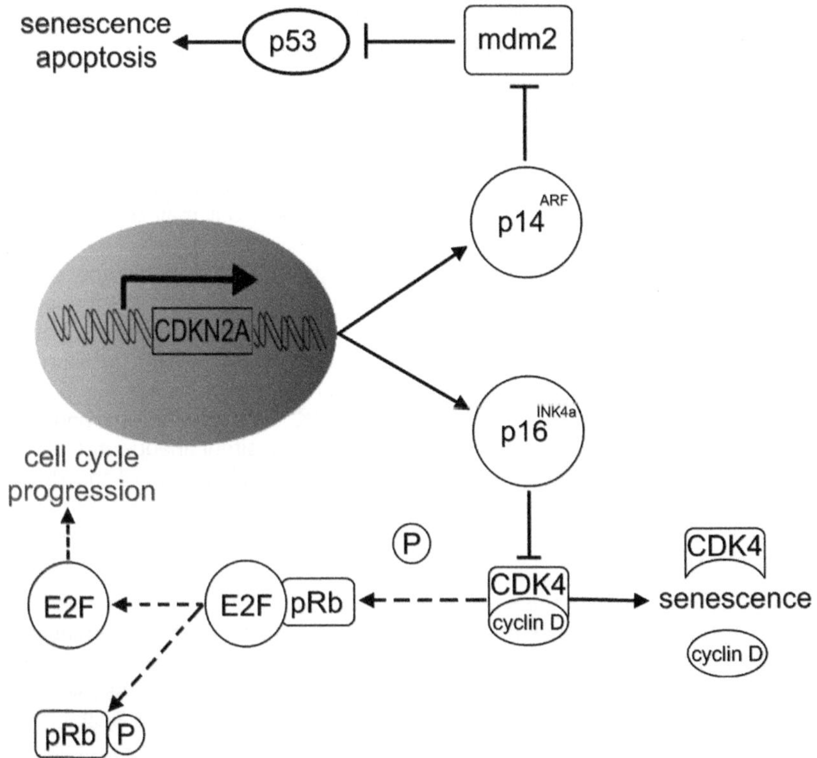

Fig. 3. The action of the CDKN2A encoded proteins p16^{INK4a} and p14^{ARF}. CDKN2A plays not only an important role in controlling G1 to S phase transition of the cell cycle via p16^{INK4a} but also p53-induced cell cycle arrest and apoptosis via p14^{ARF}.

tumors, but frequently absent in advanced primary and metastatic melanoma. This situation suggests that alteration is not necessary for tumor initiation, but may be an intermediate event necessary for further progression to invasion and metastasis.[36,40] Rather than loss of p16^{INK4a}, melanoma occasionally shows amplifications of the cyclin D1 and CDK4 genes, with cyclin D1 amplification described most frequently in acral tumors.[22,41]

High expression of p16^{INK4a} is seen in nevi, where the protein seems to have a tumor suppressor function specifically in the setting of MAPK mutations.[21,42–44] Increased melanocyte proliferation induces p16^{INK4a} and p53, which inhibit cell division and force melanocytes into a G0-like phase of the cell cycle. This phase has been termed oncogene-induced senescence. Using this model, benign common acquired nevi represent senescent clones of melanocytes that require dysregulation of the p16^{INK4a}/pRb pathway along with other alterations, such as telomerase activation, to progress to melanoma.[45] Oncogene-induced senescence has also been described in Spitz nevi,[21] whereby a proportion of Spitz nevi with mutations of H-ras, a rare event in melanoma and common acquired nevi, show increased p16^{INK4a} expression.

p14^{ARF} and p53

p14^{ARF} directly effects p53 expression by sequestration of the protein mdm2, which promotes p53 degradation (see **Fig. 3**). Melanoma cells consequently may achieve one of the hallmarks of cancer, evasion of apoptosis, via alterations of CDK2NA and loss of p14^{ARF}. Mutation, deletion, or methylation of CDK2NA may therefore explain why p53 gene mutations are surprisingly rare in melanoma, around 12%, when they are found in more than 55% of human malignancies as a whole.[46]

It can be seen therefore that CDK2NA can affect both the pRb and p53 pathways, with considerable effects on senescence and apoptosis (see **Fig. 3**). Indeed, in mouse models synergy between p53 and pRb pathways has been demonstrated.[47]

Having described signature molecular changes in melanoma, the discussion now turns to some "noncore" changes and how they were identified. See **Box 1** for a summary of signature genetic changes in cutaneous melanoma.

MOLECULAR PATHOLOGY BEYOND SIGNATURE CHANGES IN MELANOMA

The aforementioned signature changes have been demonstrated by various technical strategies. For example, the importance of BRAF mutation is shown by mutation

Box 1
Signature genetic changes in cutaneous melanoma

- **NRAS**: Oncogene encoding a membrane bound protein kinase that activates both the MAPK and PI3K-Akt pathways, thereby promoting cell proliferation.
- **BRAF**: Oncogene encoding a protein kinase situated downstream from NRAS, which activates the MAPK pathway, thereby promoting cell proliferation.
- **PTEN**: Tumor suppressor that inhibits the NRAS target PI3K thereby inhibiting Akt-induced cell proliferation and survival. Inherited mutations produce Cowden syndrome.
- **p16^{INK4a}**: Tumor suppressor encoded by the CDKN2A gene; inhibits cyclin-dependent kinases 2 and 4, thereby arresting G1 to S transition of the cell cycle. Inherited mutations are associated with melanoma susceptibility syndromes.
- **p14^{ARF}**: Tumor suppressor encoded via an alternative reading frame of the CDKN2A gene; inhibits MDM2, thereby promot-ing p53-induced cell cycle arrest and apoptosis.

analysis in human tumor cell lines and tissues,[48] in animal models, such as zebrafish,[49] and in models of melanoma using reconstituted human skin grafted onto mice.[50] Many of the signature changes occur in primary tumors, but a key future initiative is to identify additional novel alterations in melanoma, especially those that drive metastasis. The latter is important because early melanoma can be easily treated by surgical excision in most cases, whereas metastatic melanoma is aggressive and has a dismal prognosis.[51,52]

IDENTIFYING NOVEL MELANOMA GENES

With a vast number of array studies being conducted, data acquisition on a large scale is now commonplace (**Fig. 4**). The techniques used include array comparative genomic hybridization (aCGH), which assays the whole genome for DNA copy number changes; expression microarrays that assess the transcriptome; and those miroarrays that analyze the proteome, such as 2-dimensional gels and mass spectrometry. These methods can query hundreds to thousands of genes at a time; therefore it is essential to have a means of separating important findings from noise within this mass of data. Several recent studies have provided creative ways of achieving this.

aCGH is a method that allows analysis of the DNA copy number across the whole genome.[53] Using this method, several regions of copy number change have been identified in melanoma. In principle, areas of DNA copy number gain or amplification harbor one or more melanoma oncogenes, while areas of DNA copy number loss or deletion harbor one or more melanoma tumor suppressor genes. Unfortunately, many of the areas of copy number change are large, and the putative target cancer gene(s) is greatly outnumbered by innocent bystander genes that just happen to flank the target. Kim and colleagues[54] showed that cross-species comparison can be used to mine important genomic DNA copy number changes from human aCGH data. These investigators used a mouse model in which they could induce a nonmetastatic

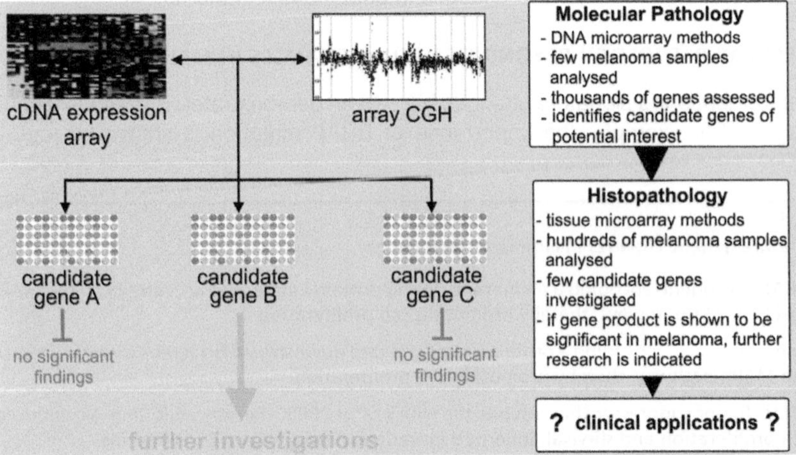

Fig. 4. Translational re-search methods. DNA microarray techniques, used independently or in com-bination, examine thousands of genes across the genome in a relatively small number of samples to identify potentially important candidate genes. The ex-pression of the few candidate genes can then be assessed on hundreds of tissue samples with tissue microarray studies. Depending on the results of these investigations, fur-ther research may be indicated. CGH, comparative genomic hybridization.

melanoma. Kim and colleagues then identified tumors that subsequently developed a metastatic phenotype, so-called escapers, and looked for DNA copy number changes relative to the parental melanomas. A focal amplification on chromosome 13 was found in 2 escapers in whom the overlapping region of amplification contained 8 genes, a manageable number for further analysis. Looking at expression of these genes in metastatic mouse melanomas, only one gene, NEDD9, showed consistent overexpression. This change could then be mapped to a corresponding region of the human genome, because in certain portions of chromosomes the gene order is conserved across related species, a phenomenon called synteny. Mouse chromosome 13 is syntenic with a region on chromosome 6p in humans, which showed a large region of DNA copy number gain, particularly in advanced human melanoma. This finding suggested a role in invasion and metastasis in human melanoma as seen in the metastatic escaper tumors in mice. When human melanocytic tumors were analyzed, NEDD9 was increasingly overexpressed as melanoma progresses, and subsequent studies indicated that NEDD9 facilitates aspects of melanoma invasion and metastasis.

Another way to make sense of microarray data is to integrate aCGH with expression array analysis to filter a large number of candidate melanoma genes (see **Fig. 4**). Employing this method, Garraway and colleagues[55] used a set of cell lines containing examples of 9 different types of cancer with the aim of identifying putative lineage-specific cancer genes. These cell lines have been used in several large-scale studies and so a critical mass of public data is available. Initially, the DNA copy number in the cell lines was analyzed, followed by unsupervised cluster analysis, which showed similarities between cancer cell lines of similar tissue origin. This similarity raised the possibility that loci that harbored cancer genes might also be important in histogenesis. One cluster contained 6 melanoma cell lines and was defined by a region of DNA copy number gain at chromosome 3p13-3p14. Next, expression array data from the 6 3p amplified melanoma cases was compared with the remaining 3p non-amplified cases. These data revealed 583 gene transcripts with significantly increased expression in the 3p amplified cells but only one highly expressed gene, MITF, was located in the amplified genomic region. This gene was then found to be amplified in 10% of primary and 21% of metastatic melanomas. MITF seems to be a lineage-specific cancer gene because it plays a key role in the commitment of undifferentiated embryonic cells to the melanocyte lineage, and also is important in differentiation and proliferation. MITF consequently is regarded as a master regulator of melanocyte development.[56]

Melanoma shows great morphologic heterogeneity, with some investigators citing at least 16 clinicopathologic variants.[57] Therefore, any microarray study that can delineate these variants is likely to shed light on the underlying molecular pathology, perhaps identifying similarities and differences between morphologically separate diseases. Curtin and colleagues performed an aCGH study in an attempt to correlate DNA copy number changes with 4 clinicopathologic subgroups, namely melanoma from sites of chronic UV damage and nonchronic UV damage, acral melanoma, and mucosal melanoma.[22] These investigators also documented whether UV damage and DNA copy number changes correlated with common melanoma mutations in 2 genes, BRAF and NRAS. DNA copy number changes were found to be much more frequent in acral and mucosal melanoma, and each group had distinct alterations. Indeed, Curtin and colleagues were able to classify cases with 70% accuracy into the 4 groups based on DNA copy number changes alone, whereas the common types of skin melanoma, that is, from chronic and nonchronic UV exposed skin, could be separated with 84% accuracy. The mutation frequency was also different, with combined BRAF and NRAS mutation frequency being significantly higher in melanomas from nonchronic UV-exposed skin than all other types. By assessing NRAS mutation, BRAF mutation, DNA copy number changes, and immunohistochemistry of activation of key signaling proteins, the investigators were able to show correlative evidence of an epistatic relationship in melanoma signaling pathways. This study illustrates that molecular analyses can benefit from close attention to clinicopathologic features, in particular taking into account the diversity of melanoma and recognizing that each melanoma subtype may have its own distinct molecular pathology. See **Box 2** for a summary of molecular techniques used in cutaneous melanoma research.

WHAT IS THE IMPACT OF MOLECULAR PATHOLOGY ON HISTOPATHOLOGY?

It is probably accurate to state that molecular analysis has had a relatively minor impact on histologic practice to date. This fact is particularly disheartening when one appreciates the difficulties involved in diagnosis. Melanoma misdiagnosis is the commonest cause for medicolegal claims against pathologists,[58,59] and there are several reports attesting to a troublesome minority of melanocytic tumors defying classification,[60,61] especially spitzoid tumors.[62] A molecular test that could distinguish spitzoid melanoma from Spitz nevus would be especially welcome. With this is mind, recent analysis of BRAF, NRAS, and HRAS mutations has produced some encouraging results. Although there is some conflict in the published data, the majority suggests that Spitz nevi have a profile of absent/rare BRAF and NRAS mutations, and occasional HRAS mutation.[63–66] On the other hand, spitzoid melanoma shows variable BRAF and NRAS mutations and absent HRAS mutation. These findings suggest several points when dealing with a spitzoid lesion. First, HRAS mutation strongly supports a Spitz nevus; second, BRAF or NRAS mutation, although less helpful, suggests a potentially malignant lesion. However, the reported frequencies of these mutations in spitzoid tumors suggest that the overall sensitivity and specificity may not be sufficient for routine use. In addition, the presence of HRAS in Spitz nevi and absence in spitzoid melanomas suggests that progression from one to the other does not occur and therefore atypical spitzoid tumors are probably just

Box 2
Molecular techniques utilized in cutaneous melanoma research

- **Array comparative genomic hybridization (aCGH)**: Identifies losses or gains of DNA across the whole genome. Whole tumor DNA is labeled with fluorophores and hybridized to a DNA probe set covering most of the genome, which is mounted on a solid surface such as a glass slide. The fluorescent signal intensity at different parts of the genome is compared with a differentially labeled normal reference sample.
- **cDNA array**: Assesses the level of mRNA expression in cell samples. mRNA is converted to the more stable cDNA, which is fluorescently labeled and hybridized with thousands of gene probes that are mounted on a solid surface. The intensity of the fluorescent signal indicates the level of mRNA expression of thousands of genes, and can be compared between samples.
- **Tissue microarray**: Hundreds of tissue cores are embedded in a single paraffin wax block from which histology sections are cut. This technique enables the assessment of a vast number of tissue samples, for example from different cases of a specific tumor type, on one histology slide. Histochemical, immunohistochemical, and in situ hybridization techniques are frequently applied.

unclassifiable examples of Spitz nevi or spitzoid melanoma. In this scenario, molecular analysis could prove fruitful; for example, the fact that HRAS mutation suggests a benign Spitzoid lesion is proof of concept that other alterations could also provide decisive prediction of malignancy. Chromosomal instability, a hallmark of malignancy in melanoma,[67] is not seen in Spitz nevi,[68] indicating that a clinically acceptable assay for this phenotype could prove valuable. Indeed, Bastian and colleagues[69] are attempting to develop such an assay. These investigators used CGH data to develop panels of fluorescence in situ hybridization (FISH) probes for regions of the genome in melanoma that are commonly subject to gains or losses. Although FISH does not allow assessment of the whole genome as in aCGH, it can be applied to paraffin-embedded tissue and is therefore more suited to routine surgical specimens. Using the FISH probe sets, the investigators were able to distinguish between melanomas and nevi. Furthermore, in a set of histologically ambiguous tumors the majority of which had some spitzoid features, they correctly identified as malignant all cases that later metastasized. This technique clearly has immense clinical potential as an aid to diagnosis in diagnostically challenging cases.

In assessing prognosis in melanoma, clinicopathologic features are currently unsupported by any molecular tests of comparable value. However, microarray studies have pinpointed several putative biomarkers of aggressive disease such as RhoC,[70] MITF,[55] and WNT5a.[71] For example, WNT5A was first identified by expression array analysis as an underexpressed gene in less aggressive melanoma cell lines,[72] with further in vitro manipulation of WNT5A confirming a role in invasion[71]; and finally, analysis of clinical samples suggested WNT5A is associated with poor outcome of melanoma independently of other pathologic predictors such as Breslow thickness.[73]

As well as accurate diagnosis and prognostication, the other key aim of histologic analysis is to guide therapy. Recent studies reveal that there are distinct families of melanocytic tumors that have similar underlying genetic alterations, which might have implications for identifying best treatment. Both common acquired nevi and melanomas from sites of intermittent sun damage show frequent BRAF mutations; melanomas from mucosal, acral, and chronically UV-exposed skin show KIT mutations and amplifications of genes such as CCND1 and CDK4[74]; nevus of Ota, blue nevi, malignant blue nevi, and uveal melanomas show GNAQ mutations[75]; and pigmented epithelioid melanocytoma (so-called animal melanomas) show loss of expression of the PRKAR1A gene.[76] These findings are both encouraging and disheartening, because these alterations provide a point of entry for novel therapy but also reveal the genetic diversity within melanoma that makes choice of therapy for any given melanoma difficult. It is hoped that effective tests will be developed to identify therapeutic targets, this being the goal of tailored therapy.

SUMMARY

Our knowledge of melanoma molecular pathology has advanced greatly over the last few decades, but there is still much to learn. Histopathologists are likely to play a central role in future research by applying their appreciation of the clinicopathologic subsets of this heterogeneous cancer to test hypotheses generated by microarray studies (see **Fig. 4**). Using this specialized knowledge will help our advance toward the eventual goal of a more detailed molecular characterization of melanoma, and the greater ability of molecular methods to add value to morphology-based assessment. See **Box 3** for a summary of future directions for melanoma research.

Box 3
Future directions for melanoma research

- Progressing beyond the generic melanoma signature to identify specific molecular subtypes of melanoma. This identification may enable the translation of molecular methods for use in diagnosis and prognostication—a fundamental goal of molecular research.
- Applying understanding of the various molecular alterations in melanoma to develop future therapies. The ultimate goal is to develop specific treatments for specific tumor subtypes, so-called personalized medicine.
- The development of experimental methods that can be reliably applied to formalin-fixed paraffin-embedded tissue. At present, the extraction of complex molecules such as RNA and protein from such tissue is technically demanding, but the incentives are great because Pathology departmental tissue archives hold a potentially vast wealth of data. These data can be used for large-scale translational research into candidate genes identified by DNA microarrays.
- Informing clinical colleagues and the wider public of the importance of understanding the molecular basis of melanoma and basic science research.

REFERENCES

1. Hanahan D, Weinberg R. The hallmarks of cancer. Cell 2000;100:57–70.
2. Albino AP, Nanus DM, Mentle IR, et al. Analysis of ras oncogenes in malignant melanoma and precursor lesions: correlation of point mutations with differentiation phenotype. Oncogene 1989;4(11):1363–74.
3. Demunter A, Stas M, Degreef H, et al. Analysis of N- and K-ras mutations in the distinctive tumor progression phases of melanoma. J Invest Dermatol 2001; 117(6):1483–9.
4. Gorden A, Osman I, Gai W, et al. Analysis of BRAF and N-RAS mutations in metastatic melanoma tissues. Cancer Res 2003;63(14):3955–7.
5. Omholt K, Karsberg S, Platz A, et al. Screening of N-ras codon 61 mutations in paired primary and metastatic cutaneous melanomas: mutations occur early and persist throughout tumor progression. Clin Cancer Res 2002;8(11):3468–74.
6. Brose MS, Volpe P, Feldman M, et al. BRAF and RAS mutations in human lung cancer and melanoma. Cancer Res 2002;62(23):6997–7000.
7. Poynter JN, Elder JT, Fullen DR, et al. BRAF and NRAS mutations in melanoma and melanocytic nevi. Melanoma Res 2006;16(4):267–73.
8. Turner DJ, Zirvi MA, Barany F, et al. Detection of the BRAF V600E mutation in melanocytic lesions using the ligase detection reaction. J Cutan Pathol 2005;32(5): 334–9.
9. Omholt K, Platz A, Kanter L, et al. NRAS and BRAF mutations arise early during melanoma pathogenesis and are preserved throughout tumor progression. Clin Cancer Res 2003;9(17):6483–8.
10. Uribe P, Wistuba ii, Gonzalez S. BRAF mutation: a frequent event in benign, atypical, and malignant melanocytic lesions of the skin. Am J Dermatopathol 2003; 25(5):365–70.
11. Gray-Schopfer VC, da Rocha Dias S, Marais R. The role of B-RAF in melanoma. Cancer Metastasis Rev 2005;24(1):165–83.
12. Dhomen N, Marais R. New insight into BRAF mutations in cancer. Curr Opin Genet Dev 2007;17(1):31–9.
13. Libra M, Malaponte G, Bevelacqua V, et al. Absence of BRAF gene mutation in non-melanoma skin tumors. Cell Cycle 2006;5(9):968–70.

14. Bauer J, Curtin JA, Pinkel D, et al. Congenital melanocytic nevi frequently harbor NRAS mutations but no BRAF mutations. J Invest Dermatol 2007;127(1):179–82.
15. Carr J, Mackie RM. Point mutations in the N-ras oncogene in malignant melanoma and congenital naevi. Br J Dermatol 1994;131(1):72–7.
16. Kumar R, Angelini S, Snellman E, et al. BRAF mutations are common somatic events in melanocytic nevi. J Invest Dermatol 2004;122(2):342–8.
17. Pollock PM, Harper UL, Hansen KS, et al. High frequency of BRAF mutations in nevi. Nat Genet 2003;33(1):19–20.
18. Saldanha G, Purnell D, Fletcher A, et al. High BRAF mutation frequency does not characterize all melanocytic tumor types. Int J Cancer 2004;111(5):705–10.
19. Crowson AN, Magro CM, Sanchez-Carpintero I, et al. The precursors of malignant melanoma. Recent Results Cancer Res 2002;160:75–84.
20. Marks R, Dorevitch AP, Mason G. Do all melanomas come from "moles"? A study of the histological association between melanocytic naevi and melanoma. Australas J Dermatol 1990;31(2):77–80.
21. Maldonado JL, Timmerman L, Fridlyand J, et al. Mechanisms of cell-cycle arrest in Spitz nevi with constitutive activation of the MAP-kinase pathway. Am J Pathol 2004;164(5):1783–7.
22. Curtin JA, Fridlyand J, Kageshita T, et al. Distinct sets of genetic alterations in melanoma. N Engl J Med 2005;353(20):2135–47.
23. Cohen Y, Rosenbaum E, Begum S, et al. Exon 15 BRAF mutations are uncommon in melanomas arising in nonsun-exposed sites. Clin Cancer Res 2004;10(10):3444–7.
24. Edwards RH, Ward MR, Wu H, et al. Absence of BRAF mutations in UV-protected mucosal melanomas. J Med Genet 2004;41(4):270–2.
25. Wong CW, Fan YS, Chan TL, et al. BRAF and NRAS mutations are uncommon in melanomas arising in diverse internal organs. J Clin Pathol 2005;58(6):640–4.
26. Tsao H, Goel V, Wu H, et al. Genetic interaction between NRAS and BRAF mutations and PTEN/MMAC1 inactivation in melanoma. J Invest Dermatol 2004;122(2):337–41.
27. Tsao H, Zhang X, Fowlkes K, et al. Relative reciprocity of NRAS and PTEN/MMAC1 alterations in cutaneous melanoma cell lines. Cancer Res 2000;60(7):1800–4.
28. Wu H, Goel V, Haluska FG. PTEN signaling pathways in melanoma. Oncogene 2003;22(20):3113–22.
29. Daniotti M, Oggionni M, Ranzani T, et al. BRAF alterations are associated with complex mutational profiles in malignant melanoma. Oncogene 2004;23(35):5968–77.
30. Slominski A, Wortsman J, Carlson AJ, et al. Malignant melanoma. Arch Pathol Lab Med 2001;125(10):1295–306.
31. Ghiorzo P, Villaggio B, Sementa AR, et al. Expression and localization of mutant p16 proteins in melanocytic lesions from familial melanoma patients. Hum Pathol 2004;35(1):25–33.
32. Piccinin S, Doglioni C, Maestro R, et al. p16/CDKN2 and CDK4 gene mutations in sporadic melanoma development and progression. Int J Cancer 1997;74(1):26–30.
33. Hussussian CJ, Struewing JP, Goldstein AM, et al. Germline p16 mutations in familial melanoma. Nat Genet 1994;8(1):15–21.
34. Kamb A, Shattuck-Eidens D, Eeles R, et al. Analysis of the p16 gene (CDKN2) as a candidate for the chromosome 9p melanoma susceptibility locus. Nat Genet 1994;8(1):23–6.
35. Miller AJ, Mihm MC Jr. Melanoma. N Engl J Med 2006;355(1):51–65.

36. Reed JA, Loganzo F Jr, Shea CR, et al. Loss of expression of the p16/cyclin-dependent kinase inhibitor 2 tumor suppressor gene in melanocytic lesions correlates with invasive stage of tumor progression. Cancer Res 1995;55(13):2713–8.
37. Grover R, Chana JS, Wilson GD, et al. An analysis of p16 protein expression in sporadic malignant melanoma. Melanoma Res 1998;8(3):267–72.
38. Talve L, Sauroja I, Collan Y, et al. Loss of expression of the p16INK4/CDKN2 gene in cutaneous malignant melanoma correlates with tumor cell proliferation and invasive stage. Int J Cancer 1997;74(3):255–9.
39. Straume O, Sviland L, Akslen LA. Loss of nuclear p16 protein expression correlates with increased tumor cell proliferation (Ki-67) and poor prognosis in patients with vertical growth phase melanoma. Clin Cancer Res 2000;6(5):1845–53.
40. Keller-Melchior R, Schmidt R, Piepkorn M. Expression of the tumor suppressor gene product p16INK4 in benign and malignant melanocytic lesions. J Invest Dermatol 1998;110(6):932–8.
41. Sauter ER, Yeo UC, von Stemm A, et al. Cyclin D1 is a candidate oncogene in cutaneous melanoma. Cancer Res 2002;62(11):3200–6.
42. Michaloglou C, Vredeveld LC, Soengas MS, et al. BRAFE600-associated senescence-like cell cycle arrest of human naevi. Nature 2005;436(7051):720–4.
43. Serrano M, Lin AW, McCurrach ME, et al. Oncogenic ras provokes premature cell senescence associated with accumulation of p53 and p16INK4a. Cell 1997;88(5):593–602.
44. Gray-Schopfer V, Cheong S, Chong H, et al. Cellular senescence in naevi and immortalisation in melanoma: a role for p16? Br J Cancer 2006;95:496–505.
45. Bennett DC. Human melanocyte senescence and melanoma susceptibility genes. Oncogene 2003;22(20):3063–9.
46. Hocker TL, Singh MK, Tsao H. Melanoma genetics and therapeutic approaches in the 21st century: moving from the benchside to the bedside. J Invest Dermatol 2008;128(11):2575–95.
47. Lara MF, Paramio JM. The Rb family connects with the Tp53 family in skin carcinogenesis. Mol Carcinog 2007;46(8):618–23.
48. Davies H, Bignell GR, Cox C, et al. Mutations of the BRAF gene in human cancer. Nature 2002;417(6892):949–54.
49. Patton EE, Widlund HR, Kutok JL, et al. BRAF mutations are sufficient to promote nevi formation and cooperate with p53 in the genesis of melanoma. Curr Biol 2005;15(3):249–54.
50. Chudnovsky Y, Adams AE, Robbins PB, et al. Use of human tissue to assess the oncogenic activity of melanoma-associated mutations. Nat Genet 2005;37(7):745–9.
51. Balch CM, Buzaid AC, Soong SJ, et al. Final version of the American Joint Committee on Cancer staging system for cutaneous melanoma. J Clin Oncol 2001;19(16):3635–48.
52. Balch CM, Soong SJ, Atkins MB, et al. An evidence-based staging system for cutaneous melanoma. CA Cancer J Clin 2004;54(3):131–49 [quiz: 182–4].
53. Kashiwagi H, Uchida K. Genome-wide profiling of gene amplification and deletion in cancer. Hum Cell 2000;13(3):135–41.
54. Kim M, Gans JD, Nogueira C, et al. Comparative oncogenomics identifies NEDD9 as a melanoma metastasis gene. Cell 2006;125(7):1269–81.
55. Garraway LA, Widlund HR, Rubin MA, et al. Integrative genomic analyses identify MITF as a lineage survival oncogene amplified in malignant melanoma. Nature 2005;436(7047):117–22.

56. Levy C, Khaled M, Fisher DE. MITF: master regulator of melanocyte development and melanoma oncogene. Trends Mol Med 2006;12(9):406–14.
57. Crowson AN, Magro CM, Mihm MC. The melanocytic proliferations. London: Wiley-Blackwell; 2001.
58. Troxel DB. Medicolegal issues in surgical pathology. In: Weidner N, editor, Modern surgical pathology, vol. 1. 1st edition. Philadelphia: Saunders; 2003. p. 139–49.
59. Troxel DB. Error in surgical pathology. Am J Surg Pathol 2004;28(8):1092–5.
60. Cerroni L, Kerl H. Tutorial on melanocytic lesions. Am J Dermatopathol 2001; 23(3):237–41.
61. Farmer ER, Gonin R, Hanna MP. Discordance in the histopathologic diagnosis of melanoma and melanocytic nevi between expert pathologists. Hum Pathol 1996; 27(6):528–31.
62. Barnhill RL, Argenyi ZB, From L, et al. Atypical Spitz nevi/tumors: lack of consensus for diagnosis, discrimination from melanoma, and prediction of outcome. Hum Pathol 1999;30(5):513–20.
63. Bastian BC, LeBoit PE, Pinkel D. Mutations and copy number increase of HRAS in Spitz nevi with distinctive histopathological features. Am J Pathol 2000;157(3): 967–72.
64. Gill M, Renwick N, Silvers DN, et al. Lack of BRAF mutations in Spitz nevi. J Invest Dermatol 2004;122(5):1325–6.
65. Takata M, Lin J, Takayanagi S, et al. Genetic and epigenetic alterations in the differential diagnosis of malignant melanoma and spitzoid lesion. Br J Dermatol 2007;156(6):1287–94.
66. van Dijk MC, Bernsen MR, Ruiter DJ. Analysis of mutations in B-RAF, N-RAS, and H-RAS genes in the differential diagnosis of Spitz nevus and spitzoid melanoma. Am J Surg Pathol 2005;29(9):1145–51.
67. Bastian BC, LeBoit PE, Hamm H, et al. Chromosomal gains and losses in primary cutaneous melanomas detected by comparative genomic hybridization. Cancer Res 1998;58(10):2170–5.
68. Bastian BC, Olshen AB, LeBoit PE, et al. Classifying melanocytic tumors based on DNA copy number changes. Am J Pathol 2003;163(5):1765–70.
69. Gerami P, Jewell SS, Morrison LE, et al. Fluorescence in situ hybridization (FISH) as an ancillary diagnostic tool in the diagnosis of melanoma. Am J Surg Pathol 2009;33(8):1146–56.
70. Clark EA, Golub TR, Lander ES, et al. Genomic analysis of metastasis reveals an essential role for RhoC. Nature 2000;406(6795):532–5.
71. Weeraratna AT, Jiang Y, Hostetter G, et al. Wnt5a signaling directly affects cell motility and invasion of metastatic melanoma. Cancer Cell 2002;1(3):279–88.
72. Bittner M, Meltzer P, Chen Y, et al. Molecular classification of cutaneous malignant melanoma by gene expression profiling. Nature 2000;406(6795):536–40.
73. Da Forno PD, Fletcher A, Pringle JH, et al. Understanding spitzoid tumours: new insights from molecular pathology. Br J Dermatol 2008;158(1):4–14.
74. Curtin JA, Busam K, Pinkel D, et al. Somatic activation of KIT in distinct subtypes of melanoma. J Clin Oncol 2006;24(26):4340–6.
75. Van Raamsdonk CD, Bezrookove V, Green G, et al. Frequent somatic mutations of GNAQ in uveal melanoma and blue naevi. Nature 2009;457(7229): 599–602.
76. Zembowicz A, Knoepp SM, Bei T, et al. Loss of expression of protein kinase a regulatory subunit 1alpha in pigmented epithelioid melanocytoma but not in melanoma or other melanocytic lesions. Am J Surg Pathol 2007;31(11):1764–75.

Blue Nevi and Related Tumors

Pushkar A. Phadke, MD, PhD[a], Artur Zembowicz, MD, PhD[a,b,*]

KEYWORDS

- Blue nevus • Pigmented epithelioid melanocytoma
- Malignant blue nevus • Melanocytic hamartomas
- Cellular blue nevus

OVERVIEW: BLUE NEVI AND RELATED TUMORS

Blue nevi and other dermal dendritic melanocytic proliferations are often considered together as a group because of common clinical and histologic features. Clinically, they usually present as pigmented papules, plaques, or nodules with dark-bluish or blue-black coloration. Histologically, they are dermal melanocytic proliferations that contain a component of dendritic dermal melanocytes, reminiscent of HMB-45–positive embryonal melanocytes migrating from the neural crest to the skin during embryogenesis.

Prognostically, dermal dendritic melanocytic proliferations are heterogeneous. They include congenital hamartomas/dermal melanocytoses, including Mongolian spot, nevus of Ota, and nevus of Ito, benign acquired classic (Tieche-type) and cellular blue nevi, and aggressive malignant blue nevus. Epithelioid blue nevus, recently reclassified as pigmented epithelioid melanocytoma (PEM), is benign in patients with Carney complex but frequently metastasizes to lymph nodes in patients without the syndrome. Despite metastatic potential, PEM seems to be associated with an indolent clinical course in most patients.[1] This article provides a brief overview of the topic with the focus on recently described variants of blue nevus and PEM and their differential diagnosis.

GROSS AND CLINICAL FEATURES

Blue nevi derive their name from the characteristic blue hue imparted in part because of the depth of melanin pigment in the dermis and the preferential absorption of long wavelengths of light by melanin, known as the Tyndall effect. Although classic blue

A version of this article was previously published in *Surgical Pathology Clinics* 2:3.
[a] Department of Pathology, Tufts Medical Center, Tufts University, 800 Washington Street, Box # 802, Boston, MA 02111, USA
[b] Department of Pathology, Lahey Clinic, 41 Mall Road, Burlington, MA 01805, USA
* Corresponding author. Department of Pathology, Lahey Clinic, 41 Mall Road, Burlington, MA 01805.
E-mail address: drz@dermatopathologyconsultations.com

Clin Lab Med 31 (2011) 345–358
doi:10.1016/j.cll.2011.03.011 **labmed.theclinics.com**

Pathologic Key Features
Blue nevi

Common blue nevus

- Mid and upper dermal melanocytic proliferations
- Symmetric, wedge-shaped
- Variably fibrotic stroma
- Composed of dendritic melanocytes with elongated cytoplasmic processes and darkly staining hyperchromatic nuclei
- Frequently admixed with type B melanocytes

Cellular blue nevus

- Biphasic, usually with a component of common blue nevus
- Extension along adnexal structures and neurovascular bundles into the subcutaneous tissue
- Cellular areas forming distinct nests, sheets of alveoli composed of uniform nest pale-staining oval, spindled, or epithelioid melanocytes
- Wreath-like multinucleate giant cells
- Infrequent mitoses can be found in cellular areas

Malignant blue nevus

- Pre-existing common or cellular blue nevus
- Severe cytologic atypia
- Tumor necrosis
- Atypical mitoses
- High mitotic activity
- Large expansile nodules
- Diffuse infiltration of subcutis

Pigmented epithelioid melanocytoma

- Dermal heavily pigmented tumor
- Frequent epidermal hyperplasia
- Infiltrating growth pattern at the periphery with little stromal fibrosis
- Dendritic cells with vesicular nuclei
- Polygonal cells with dark pigmentation obscuring nuclear detail
- "Diagnostic" large epithelioid cells with abundant cytoplasm, peripheral pigmentation, large vesicular nuclei, and eosinophilic macronuclei

nevi can be diagnosed easily by clinical observation or with the help of dermoscopy,[2] numerous variants and related lesions have been described that can produce difficulties in diagnosing these lesions with certainty.

Tieche, a student of Jadassohn, first described histologic features of the common blue nevus more than a century ago.[3] Although blue nevi occur at any age, they are most frequently noted in the second decade of life. They are usually solitary and found on the head and the neck, the sacral region, and the dorsal aspects of distal extremities. Extracutaneous blue nevi have been reported in various sites, such as intraoral and sinonasal mucosa, prostate, cervix, vagina, spermatic cord, and lymph nodes.[4–12] Grossly, they appear as solitary, small (usually <1 cm) slate blue to blue-black macules or papules. Several different clinical variants of blue nevus have been described, including:

Eruptive[13–15]
Plaque-like[16–18]
Agminate[19,20]
Linear[21]
Satellite[22]
Disseminated[13,23]
Familial[24,25]
Targetoid.[26]

The sclerosing variant of blue nevus is of special importance because it can cause confusion with other skin tumors. Sclerosing blue nevus is a firm papule or nodule surrounded by a blue or slate gray halo that can arise almost anywhere, including the scalp.

Cellular blue nevus was first described by Darrier and was initially considered a melanoma variant. It is most commonly seen on the buttocks, followed by head and neck and extremities. Grossly, cellular blue nevi are larger than blue nevi (1–3 cm), sometimes attaining a large size. They may appear as multiple bluish-gray, firm, deep dermal nodules and tend to be much more elevated with a smoother surface. Ulceration rarely occurs. Involvement of the subcutaneous and soft tissue, such as skeletal muscle, tendon, or bone of the scalp may occur.[27] Amelanotic variant lacks expected pigmentation and is never suspected clinically.

Malignant blue nevus is, by definition, a malignant melanoma that arises within a pre-existing blue nevus or at the site of prior biopsy or excision of a blue nevus or as melanoma reminiscent of blue nevus.[28–32] Most commonly affecting elderly men, it appears as a darkly pigmented ulcerated plaque or nodule on the scalp or extremities. Malignant blue nevi are locally aggressive and frequently metastasize.[32,33]

Epithelioid blue nevus was first described in patients with Carney complex, a familial lentiginosis and low-grade multiorgan neoplasia syndrome.[34] Histologically similar lesions occurring sporadically have been considered to represent a so-called "animal-type" variant of melanoma.[35] Our recent series of studies established that epithelioid blue nevus and histologically identical sporadic tumors, including most lesions previously considered as animal-type melanoma, are best considered as a single entity. We coined the term "pigmented epithelioid melanocytoma" to emphasize the unique nature of this tumor. Unlike a benign nevus, PEM frequently metastasizes to lymph nodes and can even present as metastatic disease. Unlike in melanoma, however, most patients with metastatic PEM have a favorable outcome. We proposed that PEM is best considered a borderline melanocytic tumor. PEM is seen predominantly in children, adolescents, and young adults and frequently occurs in races less susceptible to sun-induced melanoma, including Hispanic, African American, Asian, and Persian.[36] It has a wide site distribution, including mucosal sites, and often presents as a slow-growing dark brown or black nodule.

MICROSCOPIC FEATURES AND DIAGNOSIS

The presence of dermal dendritic melanocytes, resembling embryonal melanocytes migrating from the neural crest to the skin during embryonic development, is a common feature of blue nevi and related entities.[36–41] In dermal melanocytic hamartomas and blue nevi, these cells have elongated cytoplasmic processes and darkly staining hyperchromatic nuclei. In PEM, some dendritic cells have more abundant cytoplasm, small vesicular nuclei, and identifiable nucleoli. On immunohistochemical stains, dendritic melanocytes invariably express HMB-45 in addition to other melanocytic markers, such as S-100 and Mart-1.

Dendritic melanocytes are the only cell type present in melanocytic hamartomas. They are scattered between collagen fibers throughout the entire thickness of the skin and often subcutaneous tissue and do not induce any stromal reaction. In contrast, in all other entities in this group, dermal dendritic cells are accompanied by other cell types and associated dermal architectural features, which form the basis of their histologic classification.

Common (Tieche-type) blue nevi are usually mid and upper dermal melanocytic proliferations. Their superficial portion is characteristically symmetric and often wedge-shaped, with the base of the wedge adjacent to the epidermis and the tip pointing toward the subcutaneous tissue (**Fig. 1**A). Some blue nevi extend deep into reticular dermis or even subcutaneous tissue following adnexal structures and neurovascular bundles. These extensions may render a sense of asymmetry. In addition to dendritic melanocytes, most blue nevi contain another cellular component. In many cases, dendritic cells are intermixed with small epithelioid type B melanocytes, but type A melanocytes with abundant cytoplasm or neurotized type C melanocytes also can be encountered (see **Fig. 1**B, C). These cells are best considered as part of blue nevi, and their mere presence does not justify classifications of a lesion as a combined nevus. The term "combined nevus" is reserved for blue nevi in which two cellular components are architecturally separate or distinct (eg, in relatively common combined blue and Spitz nevus). Dendritic cells are identical to those of

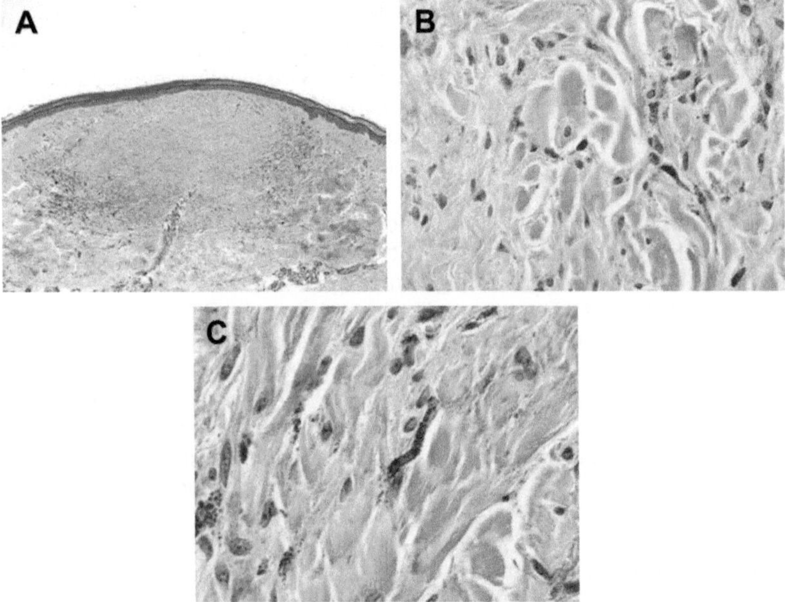

Fig. 1. Blue nevus. (*A*) Blue nevus (4× magnification). The lesion is wedge shaped and associated with stromal fibrosis. (*B*) Blue nevus composed of type B melanocytes and dendritic cells (40× magnification). (*C*) Typical dendritic cells (60× magnification).

dermal melanocytomas. Their nuclei are small, hyperchromatic, elongated, and rarely round or oval. They are often arranged with their long axis parallel to the surface of the epidermis and are easiest to identify at the periphery of the lesion. Most, if not all, fully developed blue nevi induce at least mild stromal fibroplasia.

Mitoses in blue nevi are rare. Some lesions are accompanied by variable number of pigment-laden macrophages. Some blue nevi have distinct histologic features and deserve recognition as histologic variants. The term "sclerosing blue nevus" was applied to lesions characterized by marked stromal fibrosis and hyalinization. In these lesions dendritic melanocytes are found at the periphery and within a scar-like central zone of collagen deposition.[42] Recently, a variant with extensive mucinous change and sclerosis (called sclerosing mucinous blue nevus) was described.[43] Rarely, blue nevi produce little or even no pigment. Amelanotic/hypomelanotic variants of blue nevus can be easily misinterpreted as soft tissue tumor.

Cellular blue nevus is a biphasic variant of blue nevus composed of variable proportions of common Tieche-type blue nevus and distinct, often sharply demarcated, foci, nests, sheets or alveoli of oval, spindled, fusiform, or epithelioid pale, lightly pigmented, or clear melanocytes. These cellular areas can be found within blue nevi but usually form the base of the lesion and in deep dermis. The cellular component of a cellular blue nevus frequently extends along adnexal structures and neurovascular bundles into the subcutaneous tissue, where it sometimes produces expansile nodules/nests, which gives the entire lesion an hourglass-like appearance. Mitotic activity can be found in most cellular blue nevi but it rarely exceeds 2 mitotic figure/mm^2.[2,36] The most important variants of cellular blue nevus include amelanotic and atypical ones. Amelanotic cellular blue nevus is merely a morphologic variant devoid of pigmentation (**Fig. 2**A–C). But awareness of its existence is essential to avoid confusion with soft tissue tumors.[44]

Rare cellular blue nevi feature large size, prominent nuclear and/or cytologic atypia, hemorrhage, hemosiderin deposition and degenerative changes such as stromal hyalinization. Such tumors are referred to as atypical and have to be carefully differentiated from a malignant blue nevus. Large (angiomatoid) cellular blue nevus can show lakes of blood forming pseudovascular spaces within the cellular nests.[45] Recently, there have been concerted attempts to understand the genetic basis of blue nevi. A recent study using comparative genomic hybridization studies, however, failed to reveal any chromosomal aberrations in blue nevi.[46]

Histologic diagnosis of malignant blue nevus is best established by relying on standard cytologic criteria of malignancy and observing destructive sheet-like growth pattern, tumor necrosis, and brisk mitotic activity. Most melanomas arising in cellular blue nevi are spindled or epithelioid. They typically show significant nuclear pleomorphism, hyperchromasia, prominent eosinophilic nucleoli, and brisk mitotic activity, including atypical forms (**Fig. 3**A–C).[29]

A typical PEM is a dermal, darkly pigmented, and usually symmetric tumor (**Fig. 4**). Large tumors can involve subcutaneous tissue and rarely extend along adnexal structures in a manner similar to blue nevus. Most lesions do not have a junctional component, or only rare, scattered epithelioid dendritic cells can be identified at the dermoepidermal junction. Formation of tumor junctional nests is rare. PEM also can be a part of a combined nevus. Dermal proliferation often abuts the epidermis and frequently induces epidermal hyperplasia. Melanocytic proliferation is more cellularly cohesive in the center of the tumor. Tumor growth at the periphery is usually infiltrative with little stromal reaction.

Characteristically, three distinct cell types can be identified in most tumors (see **Fig. 4**B, C). Dendritic cells are reminiscent of dendritic cells of common blue nevi

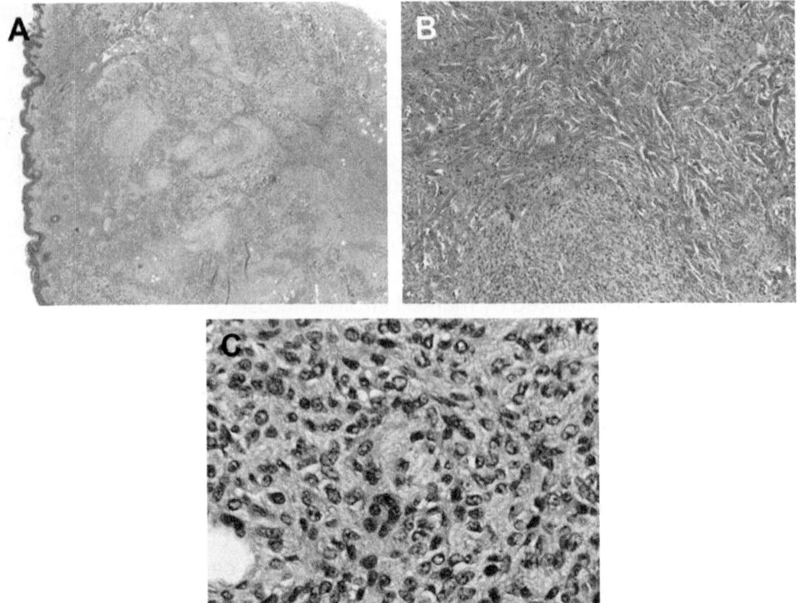

Fig. 2. Amelanotic cellular blue nevus. (*A*) Low magnification view of an amelanotic Cblue nevus with biphasic alveolar growth pattern (4× magnification). There is a sharp demarcation between the common blue nevus area in the superficial dermis and cellular nodules in the deeper dermis. (*B*) Transition between blue nevus and cellular blue nevus component (10× magnification). (*C*) Cytologic detail of cells from the cellular area, with spindle to oval nuclei with regular nuclear outlines, inconspicuous nucleoli, and diffuse chromatin pattern (40× magnification).

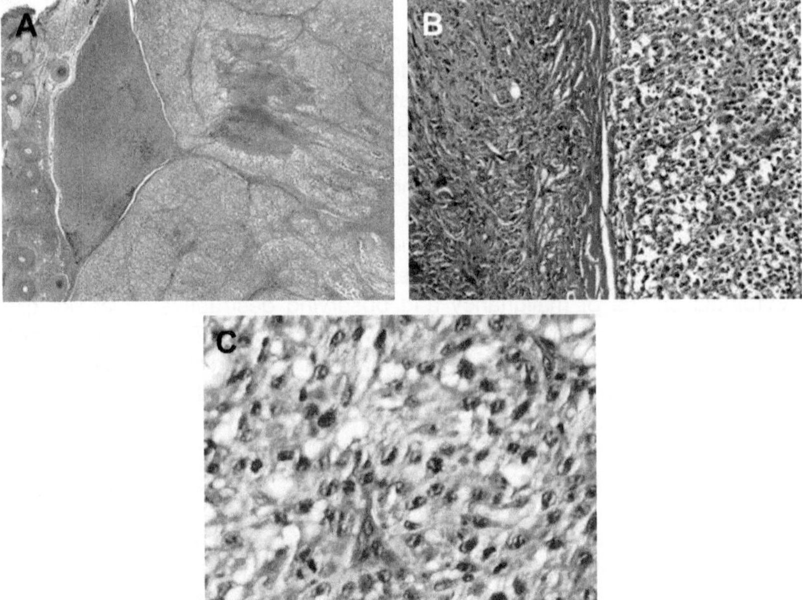

Fig. 3. Malignant blue nevus. (*A, B*) Dermal proliferation of severely atypical melanocytes with foci of necrosis arising in association with a cellular blue nevus with some remnants of a common blue nevus (*A*, 2× magnification; *B*, 20× magnification). (*C*) Higher magnification of the malignant foci shows severely atypical cells with nuclear pleomorphism, eosinophilic macronucleoli, and atypical mitotic activity (40× magnification).

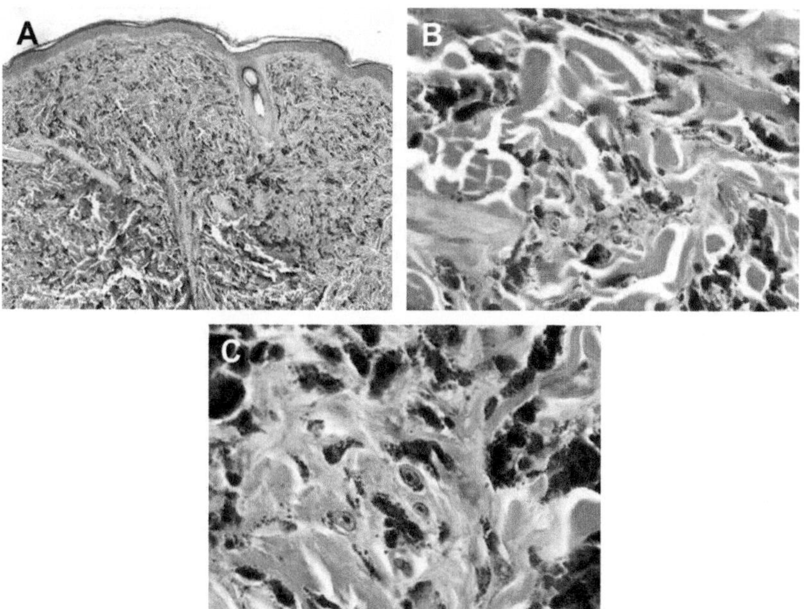

Fig. 4. Pigmented epithelioid melanocytoma (PEM). (*A*) Low magnification (4×) view of a dermal, darkly pigmented, and symmetric tumor. (*B, C*) Three cell types associated with PEM: large epithelioid cells with vesicular nuclei, prominent eosinophilic nucleoli, and perinuclear cytoplasmic clearing along with pigmented dendritic processes of smaller epithelioid and spindled cells (*B*, 20× magnification; *C*, 60× magnification).

but often have more abundant cytoplasm and small vesicular rather than hyperchromatic nuclei. Intermediate, polygonal cells are characterized by heavy cytoplasmic pigmentation, which often obscures the nuclear detail. Some of these cells may be macrophages. The most characteristic and "diagnostic" are the large epithelioid cells, which are medium to large in size. Their nuclei are vesicular and often polymorphic with prominent eosinophilic macronuclei. The cytoplasm is abundant and clear or lightly pigmented. Pigment is typically concentrated around the cellular border, resulting in a perinuclear cytoplasmic clearing. It gives them a "fried egg" appearance. In some cases, the large epithelioid cells are multinucleated. Mitotic activity is rare but can be observed. PEM seems to be unique at a molecular level because it is associated with the loss of a Carney complex gene protein kinase A regulatory subunit 1 α (R1α) in 80% of cases.[47] R1 α is involved in cAMP signaling responsible for regulation of melanogenesis and melanocytic proliferation. It is expressed in normal melanocytes and most other melanocytic proliferations, including nevi, common and cellular blue nevi, malignant blue nevi, and melanomas. Further understanding of the molecular basis of blue nevi and PEM is needed to determine if PEM is a member of a blue nevus family or represents an entirely different lesion with incidentally similar histologic features.

DIFFERENTIAL DIAGNOSIS

Most blue nevi are easy to recognize. Common but usually trivial problems involve differential diagnosis with pigmented scars, postinflammatory hyperpigmentation,

Differential Diagnosis
Blue nevi

Comparison of Blue Nevi with	Differential with Blue Nevi
Pigmented scars Postinflammatory hyperpigmentation Regressing nevi Drug-induced pigmentation	Dermal pigment-loaded fibroblast and fibrohistiocytes can assume dendritic morphology Pigment deposition in drug-induced pigmentation can be perivascular and interstitial and can mimic dendritic cells *Confirm by observation*: Postinflammatory pigment is often perivascular True dendritic blue nevus cells are located in reticular dermis and induce stromal sclerosis Pigment in drug-induced pigmentation tests positive for Fontana-Masson and iron stains
Desmoplastic melanoma	Can mimic sclerosing variant of blue nevi Frequently associated with atypical lentiginous melanocytic hyperplasia or outright melanoma in situ Tumor cells usually larger and more hyperchromatic Mitotic activity hard to find Strong suspicion of melanoma if presence of tumor-associated lymphocytic infiltrate and true perineural invasion Most DMs are HMB-45 negative; Mart1 usually negative
Atypical cellular blue nevus	Large size (>10 cm) Involvement of deep tissues Large cellular expansile tumor nests Foci of increased mitotic activity Can be associated with degenerative changes, including hemorrhage, hemosiderin deposition, and stromal hyalinization Atypical blue nevus behaves in a benign fashion. *Confirm by observation*: Distinguish degenerative changes from true tumor necrosis (presence of tumor necrosis is among the most discriminatory criteria) Atypical mitotic activity and high-grade epithelioid or spindle cell cytologic atypia raise possibility of malignancy
Dermatofibroma	*Differential with amelanotic and hypomelanotic blue nevi* Architectural features offer valuable clues Mid-dermal tumor with a round outline Shows storiform growth pattern Typically induces epidermal hyperplasia Can be pigmented, but pigmented (aneurismal) variant is caused by hemorrhage and hemosiderin accumulation rather than melanin

	Confirm by:
	HMB-45, Mart-1, and S-100
Other soft tissue tumor	*Clear cell:*
Clear cell sarcoma	Clear cell and Cblue nevus can have nested growth pattern and can contain wreath-like multinucleated giant cells
Cellular neurothekeoma	Clear cell and Cblue nevus express markers of melanocytic differentiation including HMB-45
Cutaneous myoepithelioma	Clear cell sarcoma is a subcutaneous tumor
	Confirm by:
	Dermal location and the presence of common blue nevus component are the most reliable features to diagnose cellular blue nevus
	Cytogenetic profiling to detect t(12;22)EWSR1/ATF1 fusion protein typical for clear cell sarcoma
	Neurothekeoma and myoepithelioma
	Neurothekeoma and myoepithelioma easily distinguished from blue nevi by immunohistochemistry; both are negative for HMB-45
	Cellular neurothekeoma is positive for NK1C3 and often smooth muscle actin
	Myoepithelioma and blue nevus share expression of S100
	Only myoepithelioma expresses keratins and/or epithelial membrane antigen and other myoepithelial markers
Deep penetrating nevus	Occasionally significant architectural overlap between penetrating nevus and blue nevus
	Dendritic cells not a prominent feature in deep penetrating nevus
	Penetrating nevus cells are typically spindled and epithelioid with variably abundant cytoplasm
	Some blue nevi and deep penetrating nevus can share architectural features, including pigmentation and extension into subcutaneous tissue
	Cytologic features quite distinct
	Confirm by:
	Presence of characteristic epithelioid cells in PEM

regressing nevi, and drug-induced pigmentation. In these conditions, dermal pigment-loaded fibroblast and fibrohistiocytes can assume dendritic morphology. Many cases can be easily resolved by observing that postinflammatory pigment is often perivascular, whereas true dendritic blue nevus cells are located in reticular dermis and almost invariably induce some degree of stromal sclerosis. Pigment deposition in drug-induced pigmentation (ie, caused by minocycline) can be perivascular and interstitial and can mimic dendritic cells. In many cases of drug-induced pigmentation, pigment is characteristically positive for Fontana-Masson and iron stains.

It is particularly important to keep in mind that desmoplastic melanoma can closely mimic blue nevi, especially its sclerosing variant.[48] Small biopsies can be particularly difficult to interpret. Desmoplastic melanoma is associated with atypical lentiginous melanocytic hyperplasia or outright melanoma in situ in approximately half or more of the cases, however. Tumor cells in desmoplastic melanoma are usually larger and more hyperchromatic than in blue nevi. It is not advisable to rely on mitotic activity because it is often hard to find in desmoplastic melanoma. Presence of tumor-associated lymphocytic infiltrate, especially at the periphery of the lesion, and true perineural invasion should be interpreted as strongly suspicious for melanoma. It should be pointed out, however, that blue nevi also can show perineural involvement. In contrast to blue nevi, most desmoplastic melanomas are HMB-45 negative. Other melanocyte-specific markers, such as Mart1, are also usually negative, leaving stains for S100 protein as the only melanocytic marker expressed in most cases of desmoplastic melanoma.

The term “atypical cellular blue nevus” has been used for cellular blue nevi that show significant architectural and cytologic atypia, raising a differential diagnosis with malignant blue nevi. The atypical features include large size (>10 cm), involvement of deep tissues, high cellularity, large expansile tumor nests, and foci of increased mitotic activity. Large, longstanding cellular blue nevi can be associated with degenerative changes, including hemorrhage, hemosiderin deposition, and stromal hyalinization. Distinguishing these changes from true tumor necrosis is critical because the presence of tumor necrosis is among the most discriminatory criteria between cellular and malignant blue nevi.[49,50] Other features, such as atypical mitotic activity and high-grade epithelioid or spindle cell cytologic atypia, also raise a possibility of malignancy. All series reported so far indicate that atypical blue nevus behaves in a benign fashion. Molecular analysis of atypical blue nevi by genomic hybridization failed to reveal aberrations typical for melanoma and found in malignant blue nevus.[46]

Amelanotic and hypomelanotic blue nevi are clinically unsuspected and easily can be mistaken for dermatofibroma (or other soft tissue tumor) during histologic examination. In these variants, slender processes of dendritic cells are invisible in routine sections, and high index of suspicion is needed to consider blue nevus in differential diagnosis. Architectural features, such as an inverted wedge shape and extension along adnexal structures (for common variants) and biphasic cytology with cellular nested component and hourglass outline (for cellular variants), usually offer the most valuable clues. If suspected, immunohistochemical stains, including HMB-45, Mart-1, and S-100, easily can confirm the diagnosis. In contrast to blue nevus, dermatofibroma is a mid-dermal tumor with a round outline. It often shows a storiform growth pattern and typically induces epidermal hyperplasia. Dermatofibromas can be pigmented; however, the pigmented (aneurismal) variant is caused by hemorrhage and hemosiderin accumulation rather than melanin.

Other soft tissue tumors considered in histologic differential diagnosis of blue nevus are clear cell sarcoma, cellular neurothekeoma, and cutaneous myoepithelioma. Tumor cells in clear cell sarcoma have a similar cytologic appearance to the cellular component of cellular blue nevi. Both tumors can have nested growth pattern and contain wreath-like multinucleated giant cells. Both tumors express markers of melanocytic differentiation, including HMB-45. Dermal location and the presence of common blue nevus components are the most reliable features that confirm diagnosis of cellular blue nevus. In contrast, clear cell sarcoma is a subcutaneous tumor. In exceptional cases, cytogenetic profiling to detect t(12;22)EWSR1/ATF1 fusion protein, which is typical for clear cell sarcoma, may be needed.[51] Cellular neurothekeoma and myoepithelioma are easily distinguished from blue nevi by immunohistochemistry.

Pitfalls
Blue nevi

! Desmoplastic melanoma can mimic sclerosing variant of blue nevus. A high index of suspicion is required so as not to miss these lesions.

! Amelanotic/hypomelanotic variant of blue nevus can be easily misinterpreted as a soft tissue tumor.

! Degenerative changes can occur in atypical cellular blue nevi. Care must be taken not to interpret this as malignant change.

! The identification of PEM as a borderline lesion is critical in counseling patients regarding prognostic significance of frequent lymph node metastases in this entity.

Both tumors test negative for HMB-45. In contrast to blue nevus, cellular neurothekeoma tests positive for NK1C3 and, in many cases, smooth muscle actin.[52] Cutaneous myoepitheliomas and blue nevi share expression of S100, but expression of keratins and/or epithelial membrane antigen and other myoepithelial markers, such as smooth muscle actin, calponin, p63, and glial fibrillary acid protein, is restricted to myoepithelioma.[53]

Distinction between blue nevi and deep penetrating nevi also can be difficult. Occasional cases show significant architectural overlap between these entities. In contrast to blue nevi, dendritic cells are not a prominent feature in deep penetrating nevi. The cells are typically spindled and epithelioid with variably abundant cytoplasm. PEM has a characteristic feature described previously and, with some experience, does not pose significant problem. Probably the most challenging differential diagnosis can be with some blue nevi and deep penetrating nevi. These tumors can share architectural features, including pigmentation and extension into subcutaneous tissue. Cytologic features are distinct, however. The most specific diagnostic feature is the presence of characteristic epithelioid cells in PEM.

PROGNOSIS

It is widely accepted that blue nevi and cellular blue nevi, including atypical cellular blue nevi, are benign lesions. Cellular blue nevi can attain large size. All variants of blue nevi can recur locally. Local recurrence of cellular blue nevus can sometimes mimic locally aggressive disease.[54,55] Exceptionally rarely, malignant blue nevi can supervene in a longstanding blue nevus. Any sudden changes in size or color in a previously stable blue nevus should be viewed with caution. The prognosis in malignant blue nevus is at least as serious as in conventional melanoma. Lack of large series precludes definitive assessment of mortality rate, but most patients with malignant blue nevus died as a result of widespread metastatic disease.[29,49,56,57]

PEM is a unique tumor and is best considered a true borderline lesion, which, unlike a nevus, can metastasize to lymph nodes. Unlike with melanoma, follow-up thus far indicates that patients do well.

REFERENCES

1. Zembowicz A, Carney JA, Mihm MC. Pigmented epithelioid melanocytoma: a low-grade melanocytic tumor with metastatic potential indistinguishable from animal-type melanoma and epithelioid blue nevus. Am J Surg Pathol 2004;28: 31–40 [Zembowicz AMD, Re[letter]. Am J Surg Pathol 2004;28:1115–6].

2. Ferrara G, Soyer HP, Malvehy J, et al. The many faces of blue nevus: a clinicopathologic study. J Cutan Pathol 2007;34:543–51.
3. Tieche M. Uber benigne melanome (chromatophorome) der haut: blaue naevi. Virchow Arch Pathol Anat 1906;186:212–29 [in German].
4. Ojha J, Akers JL, Akers JO, et al. Intraoral cellular blue nevus: report of a unique histopathologic entity and review of the literature. Cutis 2007;80:189–92.
5. Heim K, Hopfl R, Muller-Holzner E, et al. Multiple blue nevi of the vagina: a case report. J Reprod Med 2000;45:42–4.
6. Buchner A, Leider AS, Merrell PW, et al. Melanocytic nevi of the oral mucosa: a clinicopathologic study of 130 cases from northern California. J Oral Pathol Med 1990;19:197–201.
7. Papanicolaou SJ, Pierrakou ED, Patsakas AJ. Intraoral blue nevus: review of the literature and a case report. J Oral Med 1985;40:32–5.
8. Tannenbaum M. Differential diagnosis in uropathology. III. Melanotic lesions of prostate: blue nevus and prostatic epithelial melanosis. Urology 1974;4:617–21.
9. Jiji V. Blue nevus of the endocervix. Review of the literature. Arch Pathol Lab Med 1971;92:203–5.
10. Patel DS, Bhagavan BS. Blue nevus of the uterine cervix. Hum Pathol 1985;16:79–86.
11. Ueda Y, Kimura A, Kawahara E, et al. Malignant melanoma arising in a dermoid cyst of the ovary. Cancer 1991;67:3141–5.
12. Johnson BL. Ocular combined nevus: report of a case of scleral blue nevus associated with a choroidal nevus. Arch Ophthalmol 1970;83:594–7.
13. Krause MH, Bonnekoh B, Weisshaar E, et al. Coincidence of multiple, disseminated, tardive-eruptive blue nevi with cutis marmorata teleangiectatica congenita. Dermatology 2000;200:134–8.
14. Hendricks WM. Eruptive blue nevi. J Am Acad Dermatol 1981;4:50–3.
15. Walsh MY. Eruptive disseminated blue naevi of the scalp [comment]. Br J Dermatol 1999;141:581–2.
16. Busam KJ, Woodruff JM, Erlandson RA, et al. Large plaque-type blue nevus with subcutaneous cellular nodules. Am J Surg Pathol 2000;24:92–9.
17. Wen SY. Plaque-type blue nevus: review and an unusual case. Acta Derm Venereol 1997;77:458–9.
18. Pittman JL, Fisher BK. Plaque-type blue nevus. Arch Dermatol 1976;112:1127–8.
19. Betti R, Inselvini E, Palvarini M, et al. Agminate and plaque-type blue nevus combined with lentigo, associated with follicular cyst and eccrine changes: a variant of speckled lentiginous nevus. Dermatology 1997;195:387–90.
20. Ishibashi A, Kimura K, Kukita A. Plaque-type blue nevus combined with lentigo (nevus spilus). J Cutan Pathol 1990;17:241–5.
21. Bart BJ. Acquired linear blue nevi. J Am Acad Dermatol 1997;36:268–9.
22. Kang DS, Chung KY. Common blue naevus with satellite lesions: possible perivascular dissemination resulting in a clinical resemblance to malignant melanoma. Br J Dermatol 1999;141:922–5.
23. Balloy BC, Mallet V, Bassile G, et al. Disseminated blue nevus: abnormal nevoblast migration or proliferation? Arch Dermatol 1998;134:245–6.
24. Blackford S, Roberts DL. Familial multiple blue naevi. Clin Exp Dermatol 1991;16:308–9.
25. Knoell KA, Nelson KC, Patterson JW. Familial multiple blue nevi. J Am Acad Dermatol 1998;39:322–5.
26. Bondi EE, Elder D, Guerry D, et al. Target blue nevus. Arch Dermatol 1983;119:919–20.

27. Micali G, Innocenzi D, Nasca MR. Cellular blue nevus of the scalp infiltrating the underlying bone: case report and review. Pediatr Dermatol 1997;14:199–203.
28. Connelly J, Smith JL. Malignant blue nevus. Cancer 1991;67:2653–7.
29. Goldenhersh MA, Savin RC, Barnhill RL, et al. Malignant blue nevus: case report and literature review. J Am Acad Dermatol 1988;19:712–22.
30. Mehregan DA, Gibson LE, Mehregan AH. Malignant blue nevus: a report of eight cases. J Dermatol Sci 1992;4:185–92.
31. Rubinstein N, Kopolovic J, Wexler MR, et al. Malignant blue nevus. J Dermatol Surg Oncol 1985;11:921–3.
32. Spatz A, Zimmermann U, Bachollet B, et al. Malignant blue nevus of the vulva with late ovarian metastasis. Am J Dermatopathol 1998;20:408–12.
33. Granter SR, McKee PH, Calonje E, et al. Melanoma associated with blue nevus and melanoma mimicking cellular blue nevus: a clinicopathologic study of 10 cases on the spectrum of so-called 'malignant blue nevus'. Am J Surg Pathol 2001;25:316–23.
34. Carney JA, Ferreiro JA. The epithelioid blue nevus: a multicentric familial tumor with important associations, including cardiac myxoma and psammomatous melanotic schwannoma. Am J Surg Pathol 1996;20:259–72.
35. Crowson AN, Magro CM, Mihm MC. Malignant melanoma with prominent pigment synthesis: "animal type" melanoma. A clinical and histological study of six cases with a consideration of other melanocytic neoplasms with prominent pigment synthesis. Hum Pathol 1999;30:543–50.
36. Zembowicz A, Mihm MC. Dermal dendritic melanocytic proliferations: an update. Histopathology 2004;45:433–51.
37. Levene A. On the natural history and comparative pathology of the blue naevus. Ann R Coll Surg Engl 1980;62:327–34.
38. Sun J, Morton THJ, Gown AM. Antibody HMB-45 identifies the cells of blue nevi: an immunohistochemical study on paraffin sections. Am J Surg Pathol 1990;14: 748–51.
39. Le Douarin NM. Cell line segregation during peripheral nervous system ontogeny. Science 1986;231:1515–22.
40. Weston JA. The migration and differentiation of neural crest cells. Adv Morphog 1970;8:41–114.
41. Reed RJ. Neuromesenchyme: the concept of a neurocristic effector cell for dermal mesenchyme. Am J Dermatopathol 1983;5:385–95.
42. Crowson AN, Magro CM, Mihm CMJ. The melanocytic proliferations. New York: Wiley-Liss; 2001.
43. Rongioletti F, Innocenzi D. Sclerosing 'mucinous' blue naevus. Br J Dermatol 2003;148:1250–2.
44. Zembowicz AMD. Amelanotic cellular blue nevus: a hypopigmented variant of the cellular blue nevus: clinicopathologic analysis of 20 cases. Am J Surg Pathol 2002;26:1493–500.
45. Urso C, Tinacci G. Angiomatoid cellular blue nevus: a variant of blue nevus with an angioma-like appearance. J Cutan Pathol 2005;32:385–7.
46. Maize JC Jr, McCalmont TH, Carlson JA, et al. Genomic analysis of blue nevi and related dermal melanocytic proliferations. Am J Surg Pathol 2005;29:1214–20.
47. Zembowicz A, Knoepp SM, Bei T, et al. Loss of expression of protein kinase a regulatory subunit 1alpha in pigmented epithelioid melanocytoma but not in melanoma or other melanocytic lesions. Am J Surg Pathol 2007;31:1764–75.
48. Pozo L, Diaz-Cano SJ. Malignant deep sclerosing blue naevus presenting as a subcutaneous soft tissue mass. Br J Dermatol 2004;151:508–11.

49. Hernandez FJ. Malignant blue nevus: a light and electron microscopic study. Arch Dermatol 1973;107:741–4.
50. Merkow LP, Burt RC, Hayeslip DW, et al. A cellular and malignant blue nevus: a light and electron microscopic study. Cancer 1969;24:888–96.
51. Pellin A, Monteagudo C, Lopez-Gines C, et al. New type of chimeric fusion product between the EWS and ATFI genes in clear cell sarcoma (malignant melanoma of soft parts). Genes Chromosomes Cancer 1998;23:358–60.
52. Hornick JL, Fletcher CD. Cellular neurothekeoma: detailed characterization in a series of 133 cases. Am J Surg Pathol 2007;31:329–40.
53. Hornick JL, Fletcher CD. Cutaneous myoepithelioma: a clinicopathologic and immunohistochemical study of 14 cases. Hum Pathol 2004;35:14–24.
54. Marano SR, Brooks RA, Spetzler RF, et al. Giant congenital cellular blue nevus of the scalp of a newborn with an underlying skull defect and invasion of the dura mater. Neurosurgery 1986;18:85–9.
55. Silverberg GD, Kadin ME, Dorfman RF, et al. Invasion of the brain by a cellular blue nevus of the scalp: a case report with light and electron microscopic studies. Cancer 1971;27:349–55.
56. Kwittken J, Negri L. Malignant blue nevus: case report of a Negro woman. Arch Dermatol 1966;94:64–9.
57. Mishima Y. Cellular blue nevus: melanogenic activity and malignant transformation. Arch Dermatol 1970;101:104–10.

Erratum

This article has been retracted at the request of the Guest and Consulting Editors.

This article contains similarities to a paper which already appeared in *Trends Biotechnol*, 27 (2009) 415–422, DOI:10.1016/j.tibtech.2009.03.008. One of the conditions of submission of a paper for publication in *Clinics in Laboratory Medicine* is that authors declare explicitly their work is original and has not been published elsewhere. Re-use of any data should be appropriately cited; this procedure was not followed in this case. We apologize to readers that this was not detected earlier.

Clin Lab Med 31 (2011) 359
doi:10.1016/j.cll.2011.01.002

Index

Note: Page numbers of article titles are in **boldface** type.

Clin Lab Med 31 (2011) 361–370
doi:10.1016/S0272-2712(11)00041-2
0272-2712/11/$ – see front matter
labmed.theclinics.com

K

L

M

O

P

T

U

V

W